Strength Training for Seniors

Gain Balance, Energy, and Muscle with Simple Home Exercises and Resistance Bands

Free Bonuses from Scott Hamrick

Hi seniors!

My name is Scott Hamrick, and first off, I want to THANK YOU for reading my book.

Now you have a chance to join my exclusive "workout for seniors" email list so you can get the ebook below for free as well as the potential to get more ebooks for seniors for free! Simply click the link below to join.

P.S. Remember that it's 100% free to join the list.

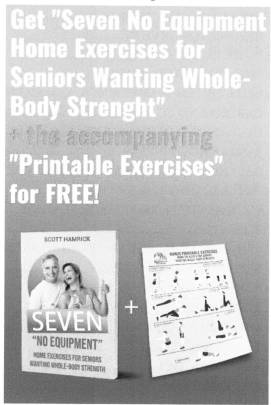

Access your free bonuses here
https://livetolearn.lpages.co/strength-training-for-seniors-paperback1/

Table of Contents

Part 1: Strength Training for Seniors

The Ultimate Home Workout Program with Simple Exercises for Improving Balance, Energy, and Building Muscle

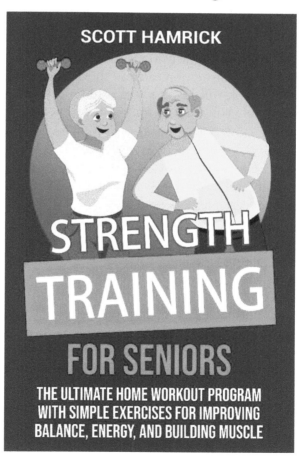

Introduction

In this book, you will learn how to perform many exercises that can help kick off a new fitness journey or reignite the fitness torch you used to carry. Reading this book will be an exciting time as your mind and body learns and adjusts while you work to improve your health.

The goal of this book is to educate and motivate you to perform the workouts and activities presented in this book consistently. Adopting these practices and heeding the advice in this book can help change your life. No matter what level of fitness you are at, this text has the potential to make your fitness at least a little better.

You want to improve your fitness because it opens the door to many positive possibilities. If you improve your balance, for example, you may walk further without fear of falling or be able to lift a laundry basket without feeling back tightness. Maintaining fitness means being active, which is the single best thing any senior can do for their overall health. This book specifically targets seniors as they have a particular set of needs when it comes to exercise. Not every senior can perform every movement, but this book can help improve those chances. Increasing your ability to function requires a little learning, doing a little more, and getting a little bit better in the process.

Seniors are those at the older end of the population. They are considered seniors because of their age, not their fitness. Being a senior does not mean you have to feel old, and certainly does not mean you can't be active. When you reach a certain age, joints tend to become more stubborn, and muscle mass decreases, so a unique perspective is required when working out. This book acknowledges and makes these changes a priority as it provides advice, strategies, and exercise descriptions. The language is straightforward, so beginners can easily understand what to do. The reasoning behind the activities and strategies will also be provided so you know how they can benefit you. This book is meant to be a helpful tool and supportive guide, not an intimidating or confusing instruction manual.

The following chapters will explore various aspects of senior fitness, provide nutrition advice, and focus on how to improve flexibility, balance, cardio, and strength safely. The chapters will be broken up simply into different types of exercise, muscle groups to exercise together, and other specific aspects of your overall fitness. Following along in these chapters should provide beneficial information, logical motivation, and easy-to-follow exercise with photos for visual aid.

My love for fitness came when I needed it the most. The journey wasn't easy, and mine even began with a recovery from an injury. I can vouch for the life-changing effects of adopting an active lifestyle and devoting time to your health. Educating yourself and gaining the knowledge to improve your life is the first step on this journey. The second step is taking a chance and trying out the stretches, exercises, and dietary recommendations. The third and final step is persistence. Reading this book won't instantly improve your fitness, but it gives you what you need to improve your fitness every day, the benefits of which are worth the effort. So, help yourself and start your fitness journey today by reading this book and gaining the ability to improve your health and life.

Chapter 1 Baby Steps: The Basics

When starting a new fitness routine, the first thing to do is to choose and understand the end goal. You are interested in working out for a reason. What is your reason? You must visualize and focus on that as you slowly get the ball rolling and even when you are fully up and running. Picturing the end goal, knowing that's where you want to be, and believing you eventually will get there can help you push through doubt and tough times along the journey.

Do you want to be able to lift your grandchildren? Do you want to be able to visit a local park and go for a walk with a friend or spouse? Do you simply want to be able to get up off the couch or sleep better at night? Having a reason and working towards it creates a clear path from start to finish that you can stay on until you get there. There's no absolute timetable as everyone is different, and everyone has a unique goal. Simply having that happy image in your mind of where you will be when your fitness improves is key to keeping your mind and spirit dedicated to your exercise journey.

Setting goals can also help you achieve more. Having a target in mind is great for staying motivated. However, it's likely you will eventually achieve that goal if you stick with it. After you get to the point where you can lift your grandchild, you can create another milestone. Setting small and somewhat obtainable goals will make your journey more productive and meaningful. You can even share your progress with others. Let them know what you achieved over the last six months of hard work or that you plan on doubling your distance by the end of the year. Having concrete goals and making them known can help keep you on track and accountable.

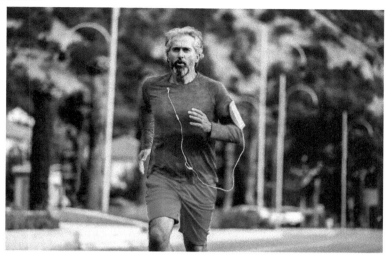

1. A senior on a run.

Fitness is important to everyone, and activity is essential to life. Those who can't get out of bed can engage in beneficial activity, and newborns still move their arms and legs and attempt to roll over. So why should seniors be any different? Just as exercise helps athletes perform their sports, it can help seniors live their lives.

Yes, being physical is more difficult as you age, but that doesn't mean it's any less beneficial. If regularly running makes it easier to run a marathon, then regular functional exercises can make it easier to function. As a senior, this is especially helpful and, in fact, may be necessary. For example, when you get older, your metabolism slows down a bit, and it may be harder to burn off excess calories and maintain your desired weight. Therefore, it's important for quality-of-life reasons to maintain your desired weight by staying active. Unfortunately, staying active gets more challenging when you're a senior and overweight. To overcome these obstacles, you must put forth constant effort to stay active, which will burn calories, help manage your weight, and maintain your quality of life.

For seniors, exercise isn't just about looking better or being the fastest runner on the field; it's required for staying happy and healthy. Exercising towards a goal will help you achieve that goal eventually. In the meantime, it will keep you active, make you feel better, and give you something to focus on daily. So even if you don't enjoy sports, exercising is for you because it can keep you going and help keep you out of the doctor's office. Your sport is being a senior, this book is your coach, and your training is exercise.

The first thing to learn on your journey is all the equipment you can use for fitness. Knowing this equipment will help you understand what you need to either acquire for home use or look for when at the gym. Knowing the difference between these things will help streamline your workout. There are many ways to achieve the same goals regarding strength training, balance, and cardio fitness. Trying different methods using different equipment will help you to determine what is best for you.

Dumbbells

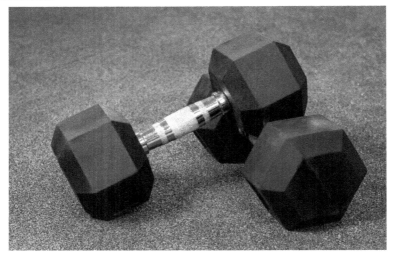

2. A pair of dumbbells

Dumbbells are used for weight training. They come in many different colors and sizes, but every dumbbell does the same thing. It is a short bar held with a single hand, with weight on either end. These can be used one at a time, or two can be used simultaneously in each hand. Most are a specific weight that cannot be changed, such as 10 lbs. More complex dumbbells come with a short bar that you must add individual weights onto. This style requires fasteners or collars that can be screwed onto the end of either side of the bar to hold the added weight in place. An example exercise using a dumbbell would be a single-arm dumbbell curl.

Barbells

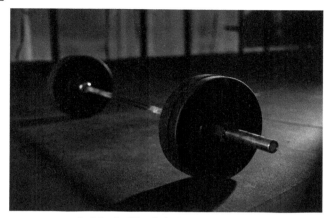

3. A barbell loaded with weight plates

A barbell is the extended version of a dumbbell, and it will be a long skinny bar that may or may not have some weight to it. These bars, like a dumbbell, can come at a fixed weight or will require separate loose weights to be added to each side. When using the changeable weight option, you will need clamps or fasteners to hold the weights on either end of the bar. Barbells are required for many major fitness lifts, such as a barbell squat or barbell deadlift. These lifts are compound movements, meaning they use multiple muscle groups, making them highly efficient and beneficial.

Lat/ Pull Down Bars

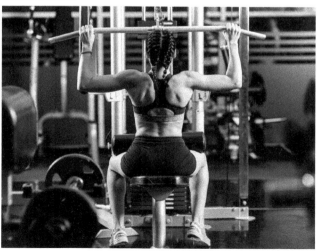

4. A woman pulling down a lat bar.

The lat bar is named for the latissimus dorsi muscle it targets on your back; this is a long bar that isn't quite straight. It's used with cable machines for pulling exercises. It is straight in the middle with bent ends for a better angle and further engagement of your back when performing exercises.

Curl Bars

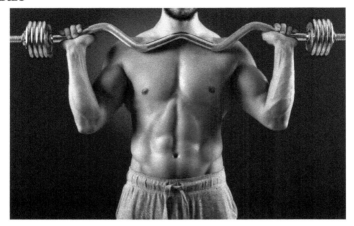

5. A man holding a curl bar.

There are different styles and shapes of curl bars, but they all look similar. They are like barbells, except the bar is not straight. A curl bar is used strictly for a barbell curl requiring both arms. The bends in the bar adjust the angle of the curl, which helps to engage the biceps differently when curling the weight.

Yoga Mat

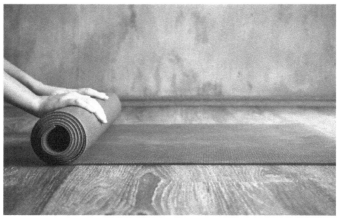

6. A partially rolled-up yoga mat

A yoga mat is a thin, usually rectangular mat for the floor. These are used to provide a safe and dedicated place for an exercise or stretching routine. These mats are often spongey, provide a softer surface, and are better for gripping the floor than other surfaces. A yoga mat can be rolled up for storage or travel and quickly unraveled for a workout. These mats come in various colors and styles, but all have the same general use. An example of an exercise that uses a yoga mat would be push-ups. Performing push-ups on a yoga mat can help save your hands from damage from the floor surface, give you a dedicated place to sweat instead of the carpet, and provide a suitable grip for your feet.

Sliders

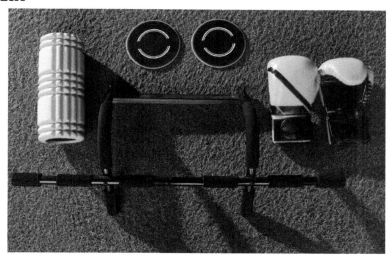

7. Black sliders and other fitness equipment

Sliders are usually small smooth discs that improve the ability to slide smoothly on surfaces like carpet. Sliders are put under the hands or feet and moved back and forth to perform an exercise. Socks on a tile floor can also be used as a substitute for sliders. Sliders are used for exercises like a lateral lunge where one foot is planted, and the other slides out to the side before being drawn back in.

Resistance Bands

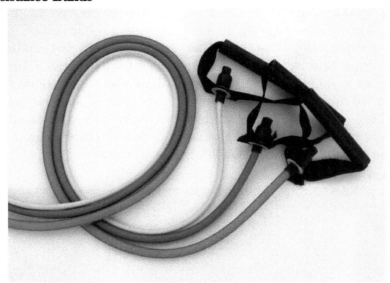

8. Handled resistance bands

Resistance Bands come in many different styles. These can be used for many different stretches and strength training exercises. There are resistance bands with handles, resistance bands that are loops, and resistance bands without handles that are single straight bands. The handled bands usually come in many different weights. The handles can be detached from the ends of the band and moved to a different weight when necessary. The handles help to grip the band and perform standard exercises such as bicep curls. The looped bands are usually skinny and wide, making them more flexible with less resistance or narrow and thicker for heavier movements. The thinner looped bands can be placed around the thighs and provide resistance for an abductor movement which involves spreading the legs apart. The thicker looped bands may be used as an assistant when attempting pull-ups to make the movement easier. The non-looped bands can be used for stretching, such as pulling the arms out wide to the sides with the band stretched across the chest. They can also be held under the foot in the center and be used for a bicep curl.

Bench

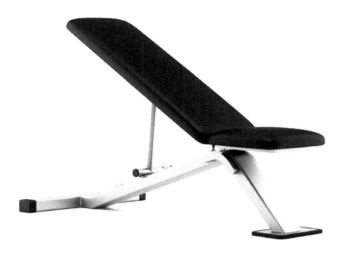

9. An adjustable exercise bench

A bench is a term used for the piece of equipment used in many different exercises. The bench does resemble a flat seat long enough to lay on that is about knee-high off the ground. Benches can be adjusted to create an incline for sitting up straight or a decline where your head is lower than your feet. It is crucial to lock the bench securely in place before using it, as it will support your weight. A bench can be a valuable tool at home as many exercises can be performed using it. An example of an exercise using a bench is the dumbbell bench press which involves laying on the bench and pressing a weight above you.

Exercise Ball

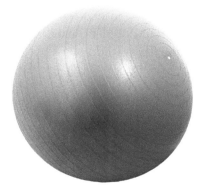

10. Exercise ball

An exercise ball is a large inflatable ball. It is crafted from vinyl or other similar material and made to endure bodyweight. This ball can be sat on, bounced, or tossed. It will usually come deflated and require a basic air pump to inflate. These are useful tools for stability as the ball provides an unstable surface. There are different size balls for people of different heights and weights. An example of an exercise using an exercise ball is ball crunches which require using the ball instead of the floor for support.

Kettlebell

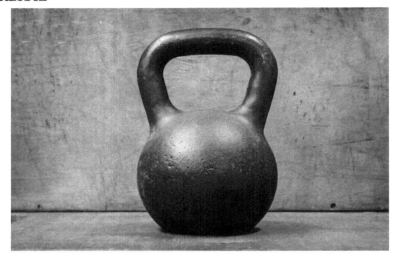

11. A single kettlebell

A kettlebell is a weight with a handle like a dumbbell but with the shape of a teapot without a spout. It is used for explosive movements, strength training, and cardio exercises. Kettlebells come in set weights only, and while one can be used in two hands, the handle is also suitable for a single hand. A kettlebell could be used for a bicep curl by lifting it from the handle or holding the round ball.

Pull-Up Bar

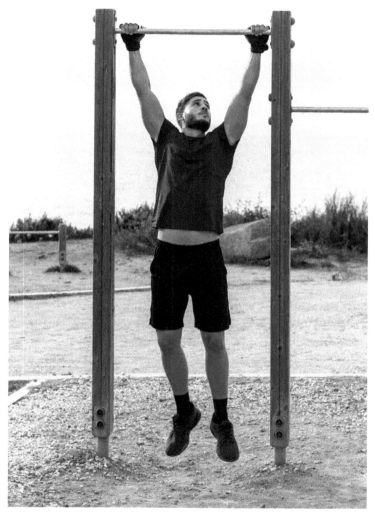

12. A man hanging from a pull-up bar

A pull-up bar can be set up using various methods, but they all achieve the same end goal. A pull-up bar is usually a straight bar that is elevated enough for you to get under it and pull yourself up by grabbing it. Pull-Up bars can be set up between doorways in a home, outside with a collapsible frame, or as part of a stationary rack or pull-up setup. Any of these are suitable for grabbing the bar and pulling yourself up. Pull-up bars can be used for exercises like hanging abdominal crunches or chin-ups.

Treadmill

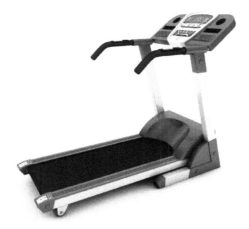

13. A treadmill

Treadmills offer a way to run indoors. There are many brands and styles, but all of them allow you to run without leaving the house. Treadmills are also great for walking, and you can set the speed and height at which you are walking depending on what kind of workout you want. Many treadmills also have heart monitors to monitor your heart rate and progress as you exercise. Treadmills usually offer a safety feature that you can quickly push or pull that will shut the treadmill off immediately, even mid-workout. A treadmill can be used for an uphill walk without worrying about the sun or heat.

Stationary Bike

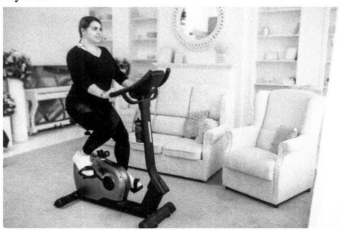

14. A woman on a stationary bike

A stationary bike is an indoor bicycle. It allows you to get a pedaling workout without going anywhere or facing the elements. Stationary bikes are often found in gyms alongside treadmills as a convenient way to get some cardio exercise. Exercise bikes usually come in three different styles. There is a dual-action bike with moving handlebars and the standard pedals for a full-body workout. The recumbent bike puts you in a reclined position and allows you to pedal out in front of you. Upright bikes have you sitting higher up, and your feet are below you like an actual bicycle. Exercise bikes can improve leg strength, core stability, and cardiovascular fitness. Bikes are a great cardio alternative to going for a walk or run.

Elliptical Machine

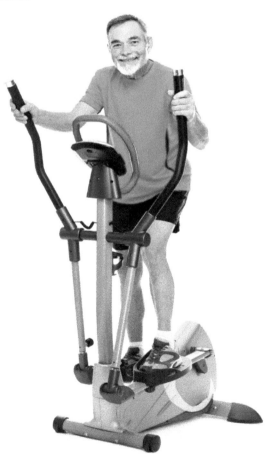

15. A senior on an elliptical machine

Like a stationary bike, the elliptical machine allows you to perform cardio indoors and without moving around. An elliptical machine usually has you standing upright, holding onto moving bars while your feet are on moving pedals. The pedals move up and down as you step to simulate a walking motion. At the same time, your arms pump for more movement and increased cardio exercise. A stationary bike can be an excellent option to stay out of the heat while still getting a good workout without the same pounding that comes from going on a run.

Rowing Machine

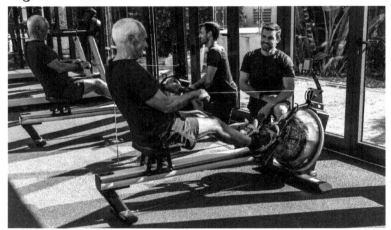

16. A senior on a rowing machine

A rowing machine combines cardio and strength while it simulates the rowing motion you would perform in a rowboat. The machine has a sliding seat, fixed pedals, and a handle on a weighted cable. When rowing, you will plant your feet and press with your legs to move back and forth. At the same time, you will pull back on the resistance cord and then allow it to retract some into the machine before pulling again. The rowing machine is a great full-body workout that allows you to stay out of the elements and doesn't require an actual boat.

Jump Rope

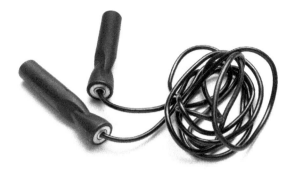

17. A black jump rope

A jump rope is a traditional cardio exercise tool. A jump rope has handles and a lightweight rope that you fling around your body and jump over. This provides a great cardio workout that can also improve coordination. There are weighted jump ropes for a more significant challenge as more force is needed to whip it around. There are also rope-less jump ropes that are simply weighted handles that count the rotations as you simulate the motion of whipping the rope around. Any of these are great for a cardio workout that doesn't require leaving your exercise room and doesn't require a significant investment.

Squat Rack

squat rack

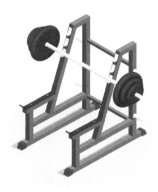

18. A squat rack with a loaded barbell

A squat rack is a metal frame that can hold a bar in place. The squat rack is where a barbell is placed when not in use and allows you to load the bar on your back from a safe position rather than trying to lift it up there. The bar sits straight across the frame and allows a user to safely stand in the middle and put the frame onto their back. The height of the bar can be changed depending on the user by adjusting both sides of the squat rack. Squat racks are essential equipment for a weighted barbell squat.

Cable Machine

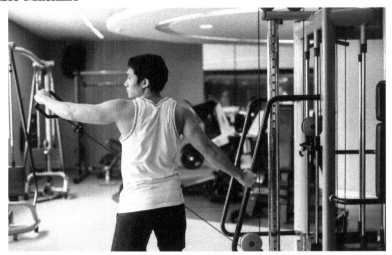

19. A man using a cable machine

The cable machine is a tree of sorts with usually four stations around it. These stations allow different pulling motions using various handles attached to metal cables. The weight on these machines can be adjusted by moving a pin in the weights located in the center. The cable machine allows you to set up multiple pull exercises at once or allows four different people to use them. An example of a cable machine exercise is a seated cable row.

Weight Machines

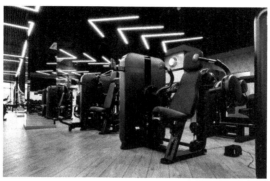

20. Weight machines at the gym

Many weight machines are available for purchase, and there will likely be many different kinds at any gym. These machines provide a method of exercising the same muscles that other workouts do differently. These machines can target any muscle on the body by only allowing it to move through a specific movement with the selected weighted resistance. These usually have instructions that show what muscles they work and how to perform the basic movement. Weight machines often have multiple adjustments to move the seat or other parts around so it fits your body correctly. While these might seem intimidating (because there are so many different kinds), they are also great tools for exercising without a barbell, dumbbell, or resistance band. An example of a weight machine exercise is the shoulder press which involves sitting in the machine, grabbing handles, and pressing them overhead.

Smith Machine

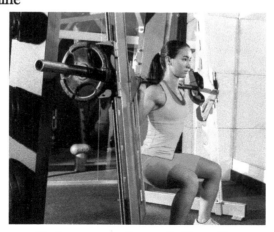

21. A woman squatting at a Smith machine

A Smith machine is like a squat rack, but the bar is fixed to the rack and slides up and down. The Smith machine is a tool that can help improve your squat. It has safety features so a single user can perform exercises while keeping themselves safe in case of failure. The weight on either side of the bar can be adjusted. A Smith machine can be used for a bench press by moving a bench underneath the bar and pressing the bar up.

Exercise gloves

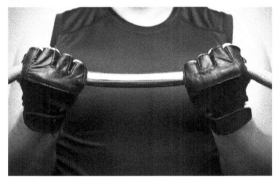

22. An exerciser wearing weight gloves

There are many exercise gloves, but they are all meant to protect your hands. The gloves are usually made of a thick and grippy material such as leather that helps improve your hold while reducing the wear and tear on your palms and fingers. These can be useful if you have trouble with your grip or frequently have pain from friction after working out.

Shoes

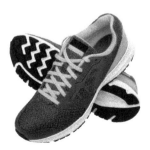

23. A pair of sneakers

You want to have appropriate shoes to exercise in. These don't have to be particularly fancy, but they should cover your entire foot and provide traction. Having the right shoes can ensure you don't have any unnecessary safety issues while exercising. It's often recommended to get flat shoes for weight training as they help to keep your feet and ankles in a natural position as you perform the movement. Weightlifting shoes are like sneakers with a raised heel that allow for greater engagement when squatting.

Foam Roller

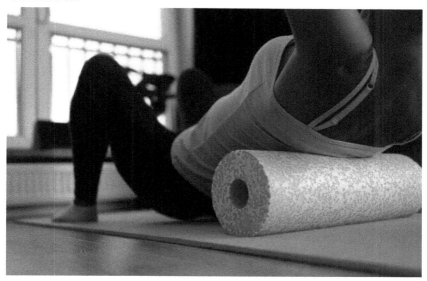

24. A woman using a foam roller

A foam roller is essential to the warm-up and cool-down processes. A foam roller is a somewhat hard cylinder though it may have a spongey outside. The purpose of a foam roller is to relieve muscle tension. It has been proven that using the roller to apply pressure to a muscle – such as a calf – for 1 minute can cause it to send signals that will loosen up the muscle. This is a great way to stay loose and relieve tight muscles. The foam roller works by laying it on the ground, placing the tight muscle on top, and putting some body weight on top to press the muscle into the roller. Then you can roll back and forth until a knot or tender area is located, pressing for a minute until the tightness decreases.

Mirror

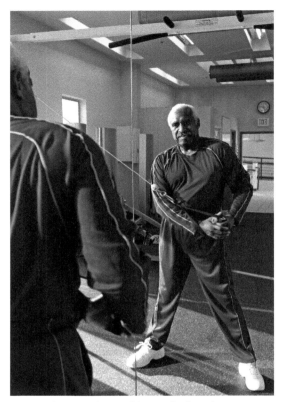

25. A senior working out in the mirror

A full-length mirror. A mirror can be a powerful tool for an exerciser. It allows you to watch your form when performing exercises which can help you prevent injuries and improve the effectiveness of your movement. The mirror can also help motivate you as you see yourself performing challenging exercises and improving. Use a mirror while squatting to keep your back straight and see how far down you are going.

Exercise Terms

A few terms will be used throughout this text to describe what is going on. Knowing these basic terms can help make learning the exercises easier. Some of these terms are self-explanatory, and most are widely used in the fitness world.

Static

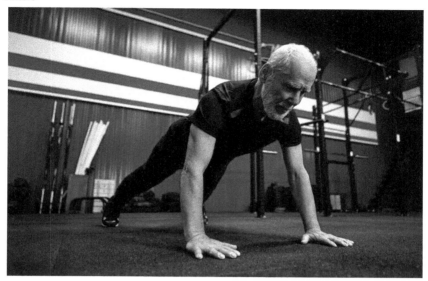

26. A man performs a plank

A static exercise involves holding in place. You can simply turn many standard exercises into static exercises by holding the weights rather than lifting them. An example of a static hold would be a floor plank. A plank involves holding the prone body off the floor while keeping the back and legs straight. Your arms are extended as in the top of a push-up, and your toes are on the floor, keeping your legs up. Holding in this position for 30 seconds is a static hold. Static exercises can build muscle, burn fat, and help reduce injury. Static exercises can also be less dangerous as they don't involve much movement.

A static stretch or warm-up involves a hold. Rather than simulating the movement you are about to perform or moving the body part through its full range of motion, you simply stretch it and hold it. Holding a muscle in a stretched position for 30 seconds can send signals that tell it to loosen up and lengthen, helping keep you loose and improving mobility.

Dynamic

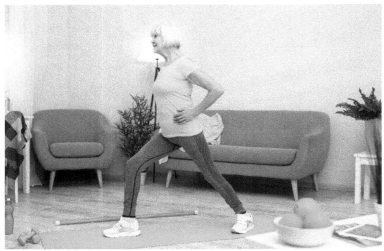

27. A woman performs a dynamic lunge

Dynamic workouts involve movement. You lift a weight up and then lower it back down. These workouts can help build muscle, burn calories, and improve cardio fitness. A dynamic workout is important because it gets you moving, and activity is key to your health as a senior. An example of a dynamic movement would be lowering down into a squat and rising back up into a standing position.

Dynamic stretches move the body part or muscle through its full range of motion. Performing this full movement can help warm up that body part's muscles and joints before engaging in a similar exercise. Performing the movement with no weight before lifting can help prep the mind, muscles, and joints before lifting the weight. An example of a dynamic warmup would be leg swings while standing and bracing yourself against a wall for support.

Sets

A set is a group of movements repeated in succession without rest. An example would be a set of 5 push-ups before stopping to rest for 30 seconds. Sets help to plan and track how much you'll be working out and determine what you will gain from your workout. More sets would be for endurance and likely be performed with lighter weight to accommodate more exercise. Fewer sets will allow you to lift more weight and can allow you to reserve some strength and energy.

Reps

Reps are short for *repetitions*. Repetitions are times that you perform a movement. An example would be a set of 5 reps of push-ups, which would mean doing five push-ups straight before resting or moving on to another exercise. A lower rep count can help to build power, a moderate rep count is usually used to build muscle, and a high rep count can help build endurance or strength. It is important to keep track of reps so you don't sabotage your workout or risk injury.

Rest

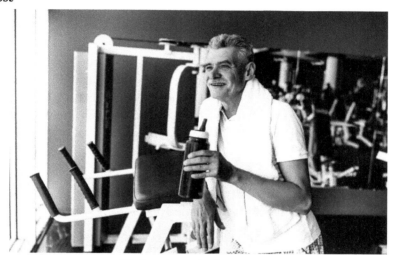

28. A senior resting between sets

Rest is the time between sets. During this time, the weights should be put down, and you should do something other than the previous movement. You can get a drink, a snack, or simply sit down during a rest period. Rest periods are critical because they allow your muscles to recharge so you can exercise them further.

Pause

A pause occurs during a rep when exercising and is exactly what it sounds to be! Pausing helps to increase the time the muscle is under tension, increasing the work it must perform. When you pause, it only requires halting for a second or two before resuming the motion. Pausing at the top of a movement is common as it forces you to engage the muscle and focus on the movement rather than just rushing through the motions. An example of a pause would be holding the weight at the top briefly before lowering it down during a bicep curl.

Hold

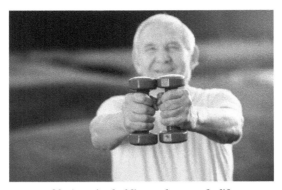

29. A senior holding at the top of a lift

A hold is like a static exercise. You hold in place and engage the body to maintain the position you are holding in. Holding requires bracing the muscles and not allowing the body to move. Holds can be used to burn calories and build strength. An example of a hold would be a hollow hold used to engage all the abs and hold your legs, arms, and upper back off the ground.

Progression

An increase in the complexity or difficulty of an exercise. This is taking the exercise to another level often besides just adding weight.

Regression

Reducing the difficulty or complexity of an exercise. This can be used to make an exercise doable if the standard version is too difficult.

Engage the core

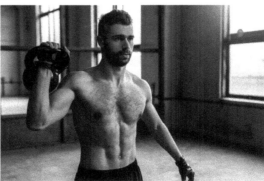

30. A man engaging his core during a lift

Engaging the core means clenching down with the abs. By doing this, you are pulling your belly button toward the spine. When you do this, you tighten the muscles in your abdominal area to help stabilize the body. It's not sucking in but rather making your stomach muscles hard. This technique is often used to keep the body straight when performing movements.

Straight Back

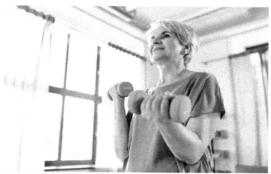

31. A senior keeping a straight back while lifting

A straight back is one of the most repeated phrases in exercise. You almost always want to keep your spine straight when performing any exercise. Keeping the spine in a straight line helps keep the body in line and the weight or force on your muscles properly when performing movements. Keep your spine straight to help prevent injury and get the rest of the body in line.

Neutral Neck

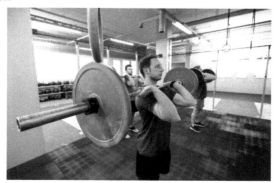

32. A man keeps a neutral neck during lift

Keeping a neutral neck means just looking straight ahead as you normally would. Doing this helps to protect your neck and can help keep the rest of your posture correct. A neutral neck is usually required for most movements. This position means just relaxing the neck and not straining it or turning it during your exercise.

Chest Up

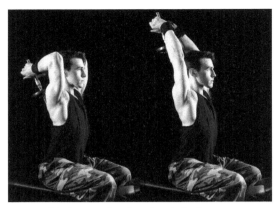

33. An exerciser keeping their chest up

Keeping your chest up helps to keep your body in the correct posture. Rather than slouching and letting your shoulder roll forward, keep your shoulder neutral and your back and your chest open. Keep your chest up to prevent injury and improve the benefits of your exercises.

Shoulders Back

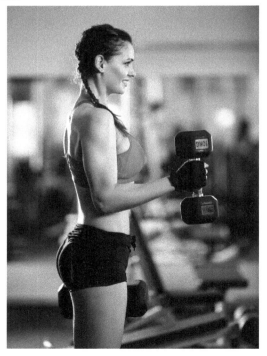

34. A exerciser keeping her shoulders back

Keeping your shoulder back can help prevent injury. Back means not shrugging them to your ears or allowing them to drift forward. Keeping your shoulders back improves your posture and helps set your body in a correct and upright position. When you pull your shoulders back, the shoulder blades should be further down the back and slightly closer together

Push

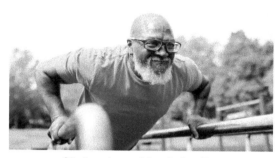

35. A senior pushing during dips

Push exercises are all of those that require you to push yourself or a weight away. These movements are often utilized together as they all use the same muscle groups. By grouping into push and pull, you can exercise one similar group and save the rest so they are fresh for tomorrow. Examples of push exercises include a push-up where you press your body up off the ground or an overhead press where you press weight up overhead.

Pull

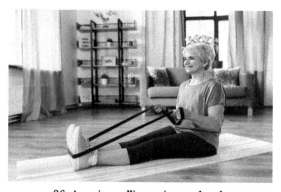

36. A senior pulling resistance bands

Pull movements are the opposite of push. They utilize grabbing and pulling something towards the body or pulling the body towards a fixed object. These exercises use the same muscle groups and are often worked together. Examples of pull movements are pull-ups, where you pull the body up towards the bar, and the bicep curl, where you pull the weight up before lowering it back down.

Prone

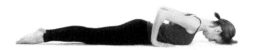

37. A prone yoga maneuver

Prone is when you are lying face down on the ground. This position can be used for stretching or exercises. To perform a plank, you will begin on the floor in a prone position.

Prone Grip

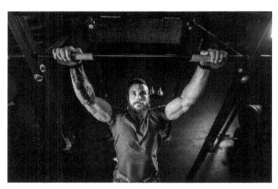

38. A exerciser using a prone grip

This grip puts the hand with palms facing the body or the floor, and the thumb wraps around the bar. This grip helps to engage the forearm, which can build strength and allows the user to access more strength. An example of this grip is pulling a barbell up towards the body for a barbell row with palms facing the body.

Supine Grip

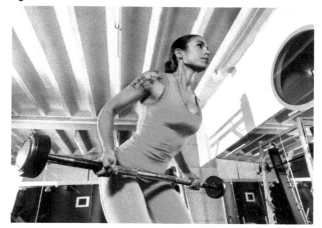

39. A woman using a supine grip

This grip is when the palms are facing up. The supine grip always brings the biceps into play which can make exercises easier and help build up your bicep size and strength. The supine grip is used in dumbbell curls as you pull the palms up and towards the shoulders.

Neutral Grip

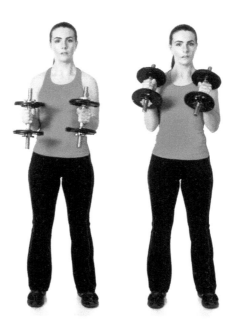

40. An exerciser using a neutral grip

A neutral grip is a variation on the other grips that can be used as a substitute in certain circumstances. A neutral grip is when the palms face one another. This positioning helps to take the stress off the vulnerable parts of the shoulder that occurs when using the other grips. An example would be a dumbbell bench press with a neutral grip. In this exercise, the palms would face each other during the up and down motion.

Chapter 2: Before You Dive In

Exercise isn't easy; it takes work, and this fact keeps many from ever giving it an honest try. The truth is that it gets easier after you start, and it can even be fun from the first workout. To help get over the hump of intimidation and hard work, you can do a few things that will make the exercise process easier.

As a senior, activity can be challenging, so any exercise effort you give should be maximized. You want to make good use of your devoted exercise time and get the most out of it. Every workout matters, and even stretch days or rest days are critical to the success of your fitness journey and overall health.

Having lived with a senior, I know that sometimes even the most minor obstacles can prevent you from achieving a physical goal. These include simple things like not getting started first thing in the morning and feeling like it's too late to get sweaty or not having the right clothes ready to go when it comes time for your workout.

So before diving into a workout, its best to make some plans, take some steps, and understand the importance of even the seemingly insignificant aspects of exercising. This chapter will provide tips and strategies for making the most of your workout and the time before and after.

Rest

Get good rest. It is recommended that adults get 7-8 hours of quality sleep a night. Sleep is integral to your everyday health, significantly affects the likelihood of you working out, and impacts the effectiveness of any workout you plan to attempt. The relationship between sleep and exercise is even more complex than that, though. For example, morning or afternoon exercise increases your odds of a quality night's sleep. On the other hand, exercising within three hours of bedtime can overstimulate you and leave you with energy that will keep you up.

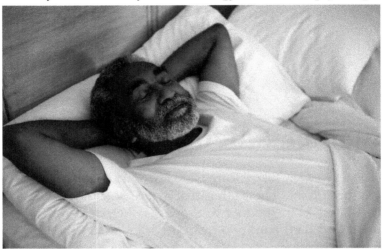

41. A senior sleeping

If you do get good sleep, then it's best to utilize the energy and positive feelings and carry them over into getting a workout in. Remind yourself that you're well-rested and perfectly capable of a workout. Remember too that tomorrow you may not get good sleep, or something may come and interfere with your workout or make it harder than it would be today.

If you don't get good sleep, engaging in a taxing workout is not advisable. This is because exercising when tired can lead to injury and can overtax your nervous system. Lifting heavy weights after 4-5 hours of sleep may make sleeping the next night difficult if it stresses the body and mind with overexertion. This doesn't mean you can't be active or engage in another beneficial aspect of working out.

Low-impact cardio is a good option for days when you haven't slept or feel too tired to lift weights. It will help get you a calorie burn, improve your mood, give you a boost of post-workout energy, and help fatigue you for better sleep later. Examples of low-impact cardio would be going for a walk, bike ride, or just dancing in the living room.

Another alternative these days is stretching or yoga. Although these options aren't as taxing and won't burn calories or build muscle quite like lifting weights or going for a run, they will still help you with your overall fitness. Stretching a few times a week is recommended as it can help keep your muscles and joints loose and reduce pain. So, stretching in the morning for ten minutes after not sleeping is a wise option as it can reduce stress, relieve tight muscles, and keep you on track for returning for a different workout tomorrow.

Plan

It's a good idea to have a workout plan. This plan can be weekly or monthly, depending on how far ahead you like to prepare or how flexible your schedule is. Either way, having a set workout planned, prepared for, and written down to reference is vital. Having a set plan can help ensure you follow through with it. Rather than wake up groggy and trying to remember what you exercised yesterday and then think of a plan for today, simply reference your premade plan. While it's true that things can come up and cause you to change your plan if you have other days also planned, you can just switch them around to accommodate the situation. Another option is if you must skip today's workout, simply push back your workout week plans and follow through again tomorrow instead.

Planning exercises can also help make sure your workouts are well-rounded. By plugging in arm day today and leg day tomorrow, you ensure that both get exercised. Without a plan, you may forget what you exercised and end up leaving a back workout out or forgetting about a cardio day. When you miss days, it can lead to imbalances by not giving proper attention to all areas of your fitness. Skipping some days like yoga or rest days can lead to fatigue, over-exertion, or injury. A balanced routine increases your chances of continuing your exercise program.

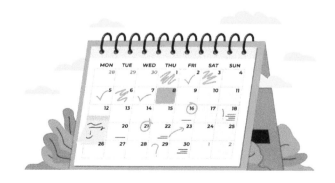

42. A planning calendar

Planning days out can also help keep from exercising the same body parts back-to-back. When you do this, it can cause several issues detrimental to your fitness goals. If you decide to exercise your legs today and you went for a long bike ride yesterday, your legs may still be tired or sore. This could lead to you not working out today or to attempting leg day anyway and getting injured. Being rested in the areas you plan to work out (like legs or arms) makes it more likely that you will attempt the workout and get good results from your effort.

Hitting many different exercises by planning out unique workouts ahead of time can keep your workouts exciting. Doing different movements and attempting new challenges can keep you motivated and help you progress. A balanced workout plan will incorporate all the different areas of the body, include cardio workouts, and program in time for yoga, stretching, and rest. This balance and variety will keep your spirits and energy high and help you find what works best for you along the way.

Setup

Planning can also include getting everything ready for your next workout. This setup is easier to keep up with when you have a weekly plan. When you know you have a long walk planned for tomorrow, you can get your outside workout clothes, socks, shoes, sunscreen, sunglasses, and hat ready the day before. By doing this, you don't have to struggle to find anything right before you are supposed to go workout, possibly discouraging you from following through with it. Having the equipment set out can also remind you of your fitness journey and motivate you. Plus, if you go to the trouble of getting your gear out and ready, you will likely use it rather than just let it sit out another day. When workout time comes, you can simply get dressed without a hassle and then get right on to your warm-up before heading out.

Keeping Track

It may be beneficial to have a workout diary. You could use this diary as a dedicated place to plan out your workouts, which can help you keep track of the next workout and exercise. An exercise diary can also be used to improve progress.

While you are exercising, keep the diary nearby and make notes. These notes can include how many reps you performed, how much weight you used for the lift, and how the movement felt. Keeping detailed notes of these things can help you see your progression and quickly jump to the next step after referencing what you did last time.

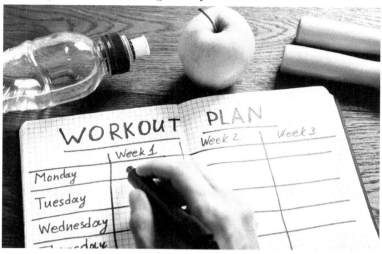

43. A workout diary

A diary can also be used to help prevent any issues from occurring again. Taking notes of how you felt from a particular workout can help with programming your weekly plan. You can insert an easy day next to a hard one based on your notes from the previous week or month. You can note how you lifted too heavy on a specific exercise, which led to you becoming discouraged or to a sore wrist afterward. These notes will help smooth the process while keeping you moving forward.

Keeping track of your great success or exercises that you enjoyed can also be helpful. Reading over positive or exciting notes can help motivate you, bring joy to your day, or ensure that on a tough day, you do the exercises you know you'll be able to get through because you enjoy some aspect of them.

A workout diary can make your exercises more advantageous to you or may make the whole process seem more scientific or official. You have exact numbers logged for what you achieved last week that you can compare to the following week's results. These numbers can also reveal once it's time to move on to a new weight level or time to take a week off to rest, reset, and start back fresh to get renewed results.

Food Tracking

Keeping a food journal can also be beneficial to your fitness journey. A food journal keeps track of what you ate, how much you ate, and how it made you feel or affected your workout. Tracking your food takes time to really master, but once you do, it can change your life. Using your notes, you can see what works for you and what doesn't. Skip the guessing and use your own recorded facts to get the most out of your meals and workouts. A food journal can help you make sure you are eating balanced meals. Protein and carbohydrates are essential for muscle building, recovery, and energy. Fats are important to the nervous system and hormone production that help keep you feeling well and balanced. Just tracking your food and correcting your diet can lead to better energy, sleep, mood, weight loss, muscle gain, and results from your workout efforts.

You can also use your food journal to note what you eat and drink before and after your workouts. This can help keep you from making the same mistake twice and possibly ruining a workout. What you consume around the time of your workouts is key to their success and effectiveness. Pay attention to how exercising after breakfast made you feel and what you ate during that breakfast. Does coffee give you the energy boost you need in the afternoon to get your workout in? Although it may seem like a lot to track your food and exercise, it can make your actual exercise easier and less of a headache.

Hydration

Fitness nutrition will be addressed in detail in Chapter 7, but hydration is a critical aspect of your fitness. The body is made up of about 60% water, which means we are mostly water. Keeping this level of fluid in the body makes sure we feel whole and function properly. Daily and proper hydration are important to everyone. Although feeling thirsty may indicate you need to drink water, it shouldn't be the only time you do.

Our body naturally loses fluid and essential minerals, which need to be replenished. When we exert ourselves, the body sweats to cool down, and fluid and these minerals are lost. Even slight dehydration can lead to feelings of fatigue or overheating. When exercising, you don't want to experience either of these as it will slow your workout and could lead to injury or other consequences.

Athletes need to drink a lot more water as they exert their bodies and lose fluid more regularly. Since you are an athlete with a regular exercise program and fitness goals, you need to be more attentive to your hydration.

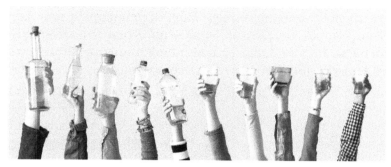
44. Various bottles of water

You should drink between 9 and 13 cups of water daily, regardless of any other circumstances. Keeping up your fluids can have many benefits, such as reducing joint pain, boosting energy, and improving sleep. Staying hydrated is as simple as drinking water throughout the day. Don't save your water consumption for only around your workout. Keep it going before, during, and after so you never have to deal with any adverse side effects of being dehydrated.

One practical idea is to get a large bottle or two of water and keep them filled and in the fridge or with you throughout the day. Having these ready to go ahead of time makes it easy to simply sip as you go and get back to what you are doing. This strategy also benefits from planning ahead to make your life easier. It's also wise to always have a drink nearby during your workout, as you will likely feel thirsty.

There are multiple options for getting your daily fluid in but having plain water or water with electrolytes is especially beneficial to those working out. Electrolytes are the minerals the body loses through sweating that need to be replaced. Electrolyte drinks, such as Gatorade, have these minerals alongside the water. Plan and take your water intake seriously, as it can make or break your workout plans.

Stretching

Stretching is a powerful practice for everyday wellness. It's something small you can do regularly to keep your muscles loose, relieve pain, reduce stress, and maintain joint health. Stretching out a muscle for 30 seconds to 1 minute has been found to relieve its tension. The relief can extend to pain the tightness is causing, general stress you are experiencing, and the strain the tightened muscles are putting on your joints.

Stretching in the morning can help wake up your body and leave you feeling good afterward. This practice can positively impact the rest of your day, both mentally and physically. After stretching, you may be able to safely bend over to pet the cat or pick up a pen you dropped without experiencing pain. Stretching is recommended multiple times a week as it can keep these positive benefits of stretching going.

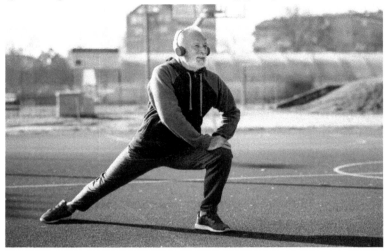

45. A senior man stretching

Stretching is also widely used by athletes and exercisers. You may end up with some tight muscles after you lift weights. Regardless, you just exerted a lot of energy and used the muscle more than it is used to in a repetitive movement. Stretching the muscles you exercised after using them can help relieve the tension you likely built up. So, a stretch post-workout can help cool your muscles down and make them feel a little more relaxed and normal after being exerted.

Stretching post-workout can also increase circulation and relieve the buildup of lactic acid, which can lead to muscle soreness. After you exert a muscle, lactic acid gathers and can lead to pain as your recover the next day or two. Stretching can help reduce this soreness before it even starts.

Stretching also improves range of motion and flexibility after your workout. You can prevent an injury from occurring simply by stretching out the muscles you just worked. This practice can also improve your overall flexibility over time. This increased flexibility reduces the risk of injury while improving your muscles' ability to stretch and contract the next time you exercise.

Maintenance Stretching

Stretching can also be used on days you aren't going to exercise. The benefits of stretching extend beyond just post-exercise. Stretching can help wake you up and get the blood pumping in the morning, and it can help calm you down and relieve stress at the end of a long day. You can even schedule a lengthy stretching section as your workout for the day. Some days you'll be too tired to exercise or know you have a big workout coming the following day; on these days, it would be a good idea to stretch to stay dedicated to your plan. It's best on these days to hit 3-5 general stretches or target an area you know needs some focus from the previous day or will be heavily used the next day.

Yoga

Yoga is like stretching. Yoga combines breathing, stretching, mindfulness, and strength to create a unique physical and mental experience. Yoga can help rejuvenate you on an off day during your workout week. After a yoga session, you may be sweaty and feel like you've exerted yourself. However, you also will have helped to ease your stress, improve stability, and stretch out your muscles and joints.

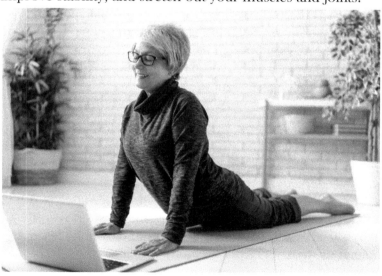

46. A senior practicing yoga

There are many yoga movements and focuses, and they all provide plenty of benefits. Yoga can be difficult, though, as it requires focus, patience, and flexibility. If you aren't flexible, practicing yoga and keeping up with your stretching can help improve it over time. Yoga exercises work as a supplement to your other strength and cardio exercising. Doing yoga regularly around these workouts improves your ability to continue doing them and reduces your chances of injury.

In yoga, focusing on breathing as you slowly move and stretch helps to calm you and can even allow you to sink deeper into the stretches. The breathing aspect of yoga and the powerful way it makes you feel combined with the movements is why yoga is often considered a spiritual practice. Therefore, yoga gets put into its own category as it is just as much about connection and calm as it is about building strength.

Yoga is lower impact as it doesn't require pounding your feet, jumping around, or lifting heavy weights. Yoga simply uses body weight and puts the body parts through their full range of motion. You will get into a position by stretching or easing into it, hold that position and focus on proper breathing before coming back out of it. This process awakens the body and mind and leaves you feeling more flexible afterward.

Though you may not be able to get into the full pose the yoga movements ask for, simply attempting them still provides benefits. Eventually, you will build up the ability to sink deeper into them for even greater benefit. For this reason, yoga requires patience and is just as challenging for some as weightlifting or running. The many benefits of yoga, though, are reason enough to attempt it regularly. Schedule a yoga day at least once a week when you feel you want a change of pace or will need a body-rejuvenating session.

Rest Periods

Once you begin working out, you must not forget your rest periods. Exercise such as weightlifting requires you to exert energy to raise the weight. Once you've raised and lowered weight multiple times, that energy gets somewhat depleted. Attempting to continue to lift the weight at this point can be detrimental to your progress. Instead, after performing ten repetitions, you should put the weight down for a short rest. Rest periods are usually 30 seconds to 1 minute long and will be used frequently throughout your workout.

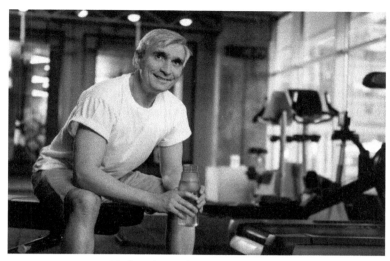
47. A senior resting during a workout

During the rest, the most important thing is to utilize the time wisely. In a rest period, you should do whatever you feel you need to recover your breath and energy before attempting to perform the movement again. You can get a drink, walk around the room, or just sit down during your rest period. This time is meant to reset your mind and muscles so you can put them through more effective work.

The goal of the rest period is to catch your breath enough so that you can do more exercise without calming down past the point of wanting more activity. When you work out, your body and muscle get into a zone where they know they are exerting energy. Too long of rest may snap you out of this and end your workout prematurely or lead to an injury. Take a rest, and be sure you feel a slight recovery before jumping back in and lifting that weight again.

Utilizing the rest period can power you through the next set of repetitions. It can help make your workout more efficient by allowing you to lift more repeatedly with regained energy. Rest periods can also help you reduce your chances of over-exertion. Lifting for too long without rest may overtax a muscle or overfatigue yourself, hindering recovery. You don't want to sabotage your workout, so stick to the plan and be sure to get rest during your activity.

Focus

It's essential to focus on your posture, breathing, and muscles as you exercise. Keeping your mind connected to the exercise at hand can make it more effective and help reduce the risk of injury. When you are actively concentrating on what you are doing, you will be able to feel when your posture is incorrect or when you are about to drop a weight from fatigue.

Simply hurrying through the motions of the workout may seem like a shortcut, but it's not. It does help to be present and pay attention to your breathing and body during exertion. You don't want to waste your time by rushing or only giving partial effort, and you don't want to end up sidelined with an injury from lack of focus. Having your exercises, repetitions, and sets written and on hand for reference can help you ensure your mind is on the activity and not trying to determine what workout you will choose next.

Stretches & Warm-ups

Use these stretches to calm down or loosen up after a workout or long day; these each focus on a specific muscle or muscle group. These stretches can all be done together or grouped into targeted stretching sessions.

Legs

Wall Stretch

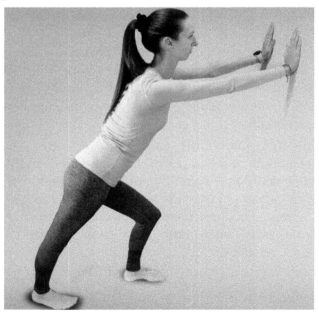

48. A woman using a wall stretch

This stretch will help to stretch the calf muscles. This stretch would be a good idea after a run, bike session, or leg day.

1. Find a sturdy wall or area you can press your whole weight against.

2. Fully extend your arms and place your palms on the wall at shoulder height and width.

3. Stagger your legs, so one is in front of the other. Be sure to keep your back straight and your neck neutral.

4. Your front leg should be bent at the knee with the foot planted flat on the floor.

5. Your back leg should be slightly behind you with your knee straight and your foot planted flat on the floor.

6. Bend at the elbows and lower yourself in towards the wall. Feel the stretch on the backside of your rear leg. Your feet should stay planted on the floor, and your back leg should remain straight.

7. Hold the stretch for 30 seconds to 1 minute. Press with your palms and straighten your arms back out.

8. Switch legs and Repeat on the other side.

Quadriceps and Hip Flexor Floor Stretch

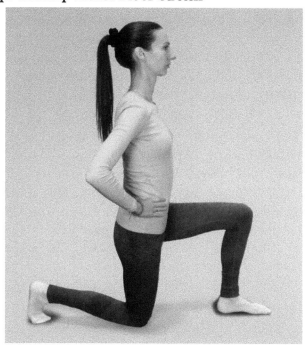

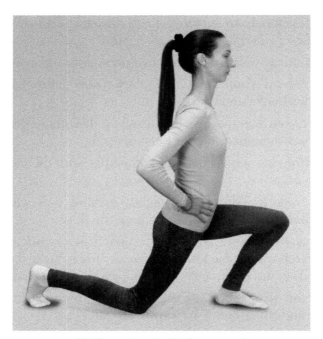
49. Illustration of a hip flexor stretch

This stretch will loosen up the quadriceps and hip flexor muscles on the front of the thigh. This stretch is a good choice after a run or squat day.

1) Get into a kneeling position on the floor and keep your back straight, chest up, shoulders back, and neck neutral.

2) Your right leg should be out in front of you. Plant the foot flat on the floor and bend the knee to 90 degrees.

3) Your left knee should be on the ground, and your lower leg extended behind you. Your left thigh should be directly below and in line with your body.

4) Exhale and drift forward with your hips. This should move your right knee forward over your right foot, and your left thigh should also drift forward so that it is no longer in a straight line. When you feel a stretch in your left thigh, pause and hold the stretch for 30 seconds.

5) Inhale and pull back so that your legs are straight again.

6) Switch legs and repeat.

Hamstring Stretch

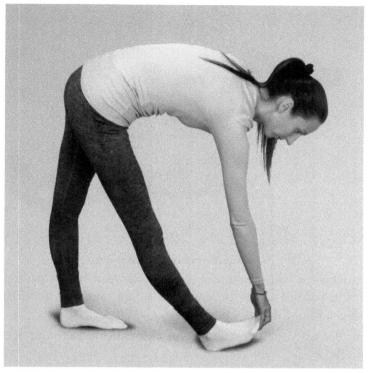

50. A woman performing a hamstring stretch

This stretch will help to loosen up the muscles on the back of the thigh. This should be used after deadlifts, leg day, or cardio (like a bike ride).

1) Stand with your back straight, chest up, shoulders back, and neck neutral.

2) Put your right foot forward and lift your foot so that only the heel is on the ground. Keep this leg extended and straight.

3) Keep your left foot planted; you can bend the knee slightly. Push your left hip out and back.

4) Keeping your back straight, breathe in and bend at the hips and lower down toward your right foot. You can reach down with your arms towards the foot as you lower. When you feel the stretch in the right hamstring, hold the position there for 30 seconds.

5) Exhale and lift back up into the starting position.

6) Switch legs and repeat.

Glute Stretch

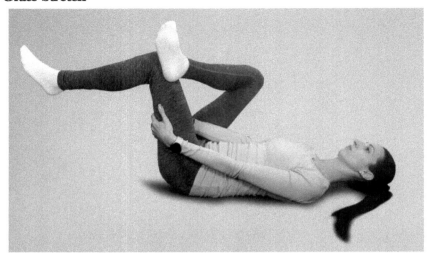

51. A woman performs a glute stretch

This movement will relieve the tightness in your buttocks. This stretch can help with painful knees or lower back pain and is a good option for after leg day, a bike ride, or squatting.

1) Lie flat on your back and bend your knees. Let your feet rest on the floor

2) Cross the right leg over the left leg. Your right foot should be on your left knee.

3) Reach under your left leg on either side and grab the back of your thigh. Exhale and bring both legs up and towards your chest. Stop when you feel a stretch in your buttock. Hold this position for sec seconds.

4) Inhale and lower your legs back down.

5) Switch legs and repeat.

Butterfly Stretch

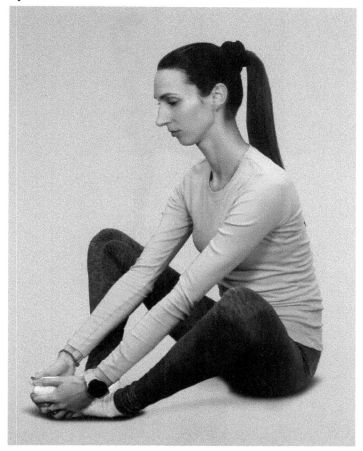

52. A woman performs a butterfly stretch

This stretch will loosen up tight inner thighs and should be used after leg day or bike rides.

1) Sit with your back straight, chest up, shoulders back, and neck neutral.

2) Bend your knees and bring the feet together in front of you so the bottoms are touching.

3) Grab onto both feet. Exhale and bend forward, keeping your back straight. You will feel a stretch on the inside of your thighs. Hold this position for 30 seconds

4) Inhale and come up from the stretch to the starting position.

5) Switch legs and repeat.

Leg Swings

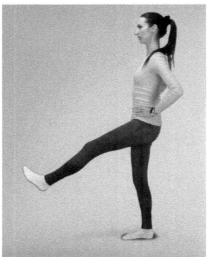

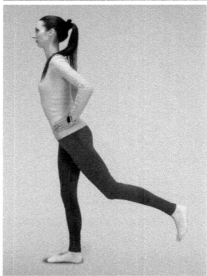

53. A woman performs leg swings

1) Stand with feet about hip-width apart and arms out to your sides or holding a wall or chair.

2) Swing your left leg keeping the keep extended back behind you, and then forward and in front of you. Continue this for 5 full swings.

3) Switch legs and repeat.

Lateral Leg Swings

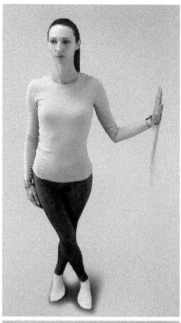

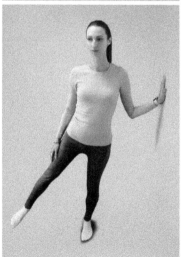

54. A woman performs lateral leg swings

1) Stand with feet close together and arms out to your sides
2) Swing the right leg out and then across to the left in front of the left leg. Continue this movement for 5 swings.
3) Switch legs and repeat.

IT Band Stretch

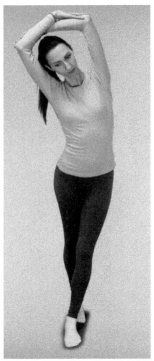

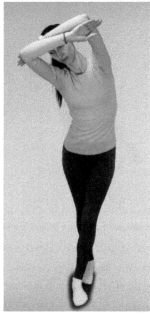

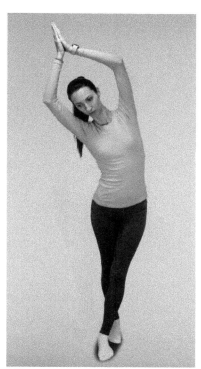

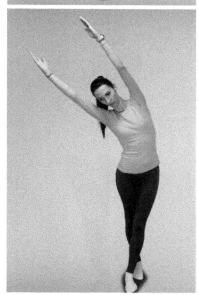

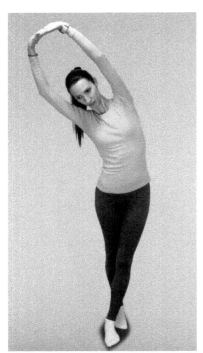

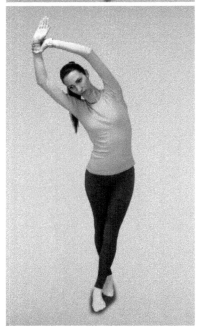

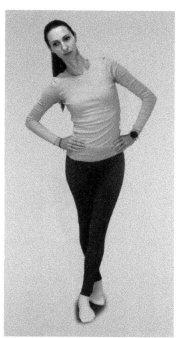

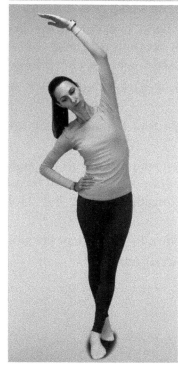

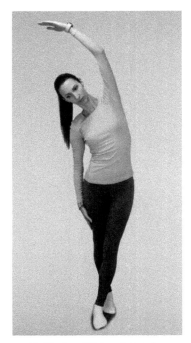

55. Various IT band stretches

The IT or iliotibial band is a connective band that goes down the outside the thigh. It can become tight and restrict movement in the leg, This stretch should be used weekly or after a long cardio session.

Stand with your back straight, chest up, shoulders back, and neck neutral.

Cross the right foot behind the left and try to keep both feet planted.

Reach up over your head with the right arm. Exhale and lean to the left. Push your hip out as you lean over. You should feel a stretch on the outside of your leg. Hold this position for 30 seconds.

Inhale and return to the upright position.

Switch legs and repeat.

Supine Twist

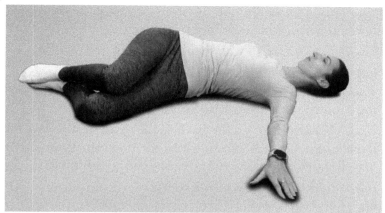

56. An illustration of a supine twist

This stretch will help with back flexibility, and it will relieve tension in the lower back and hips. Use this after a back day, abs day, or long cardio session.

1) Lie on your back with your knees bent and feet flat on the floor.
2) Keep your back flat. Exhale and slowly rotate your hips and lower your legs the way they are down to the left. You will feel a stretch along the way. Hold this position for 15-30 seconds.
3) Inhale and return to the starting position.
4) Exhale before repeating on the other side.

Knee-to-Chest

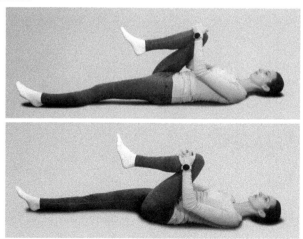

57. A woman performs a knee-to-chest stretch

This stretch will help loosen up the muscle of the lower back as well as the glutes. This stretch should be used regularly or after back day, especially when performing deadlifts.

1) Lie flat on your back with your knees bent and feet flat.

2) Extend your right knee straight out with the heel on the floor and your toes pointing towards the ceiling. Keep your hips down, and your spine lengthened.

3) Grab your left knee on the back of the thigh or the top of the shin. Exhale and bring it up and into your chest; when you feel the stretch, hold this position for 30 seconds to 1 minute.

4) Inhale ad lower your leg back down.

5) Switch legs and repeat.

Cat-Cow

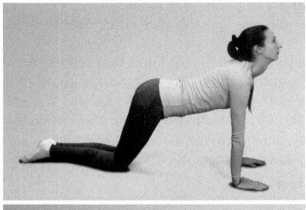

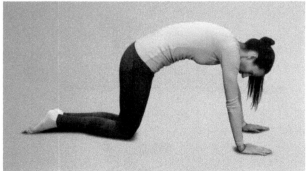

58. A woman performs a cat-cow stretch

This stretch will loosen up the shoulders, neck, chest, and back, and it will help with correcting posture by invigorating your spine.

1) Get onto all fours on the floor with your palms flat on the floor directly below your shoulders.

2) Inhale and raise up your head and look at the ceiling. At the same time, let your belly hang low and fill with air. Your tailbone will also raise up into the air.

3) Exhale and arch your spine, tuck your tailbone in, and bring toward chin down to your chest.

4) Continue to switch between the two positions while breathing for at least 1 minute.

Upper Trapezius Stretch

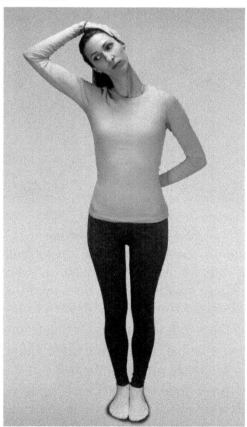

59. A woman stretching his trapezius

This stretch can reduce tension in the neck and the muscle at the top of your back and can help relieve stress. Use this stretch to loosen up after a back day.

1) Stand with your back straight, chest up, shoulders back, and neck neutral.

2) Place your left hand on your lower back, with the top of your hands touching your skin.

3) Place your right hand on your head, grabbing the left side.

4) Exhale and gently pull your neck over to the right side until you feel a stretch. Hold this position for 30 seconds.

5) Inhale and release your head back to neutral.

6) Switch your hands and stretch the other side.

Lat Ball Stretch

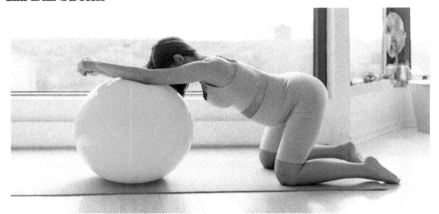

60. A woman stretching her lats

This stretch requires you to use your exercise ball. It is an excellent stretch for your lat muscles. They are located on either side of the back below the armpit. These muscles are the ones used for significant pulling motions such as pull-ups or rowing. Use this stretch after *back day.*

1) Begin on all fours with the exercise ball in front of you.

2) Place the exercise ball under your right elbow and extend your arm, so it rests straight on top of the ball.

3) Exhale and press your hips backward while putting pressure on the ball with your arm. Try to focus on stretching the lats on either side of your back. Once you feel the stretch, hold this position for 1 minute.

4) Inhale and return to the starting position.

5) Move the ball over to the left arm and repeat.

Abdominal Twist

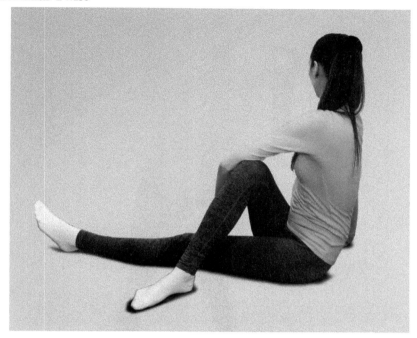

61. A woman performing an abdominal twist

This stretch is beneficial to multiple areas of the body. Use this to stretch and wake up the neck, shoulders, abdominals, hips, and back. Perform this stretch regularly or after back or ab workout days.

1) Sit with your back straight, chest up, shoulders back, and neck neutral.

2) Extend your legs straight out in front of you with your toes pointing to the ceiling.

3) Bend your right knee and place your foot outside your left thigh.

4) Extend your left arm and place it outside your right thigh.

5) Put your right hand behind your body with the fingers pointing away from your body.

6) Exhale and slowly twist the body around to the right side. As you turn, look over your right shoulder. Hold this position for 30 seconds to 1 minute.

7) Switch legs and repeat on the other side.

Side Stretch

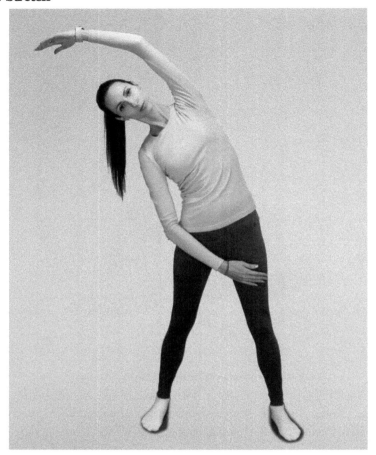

62. A woman performing a side stretch

This stretch will stretch out and awaken the muscles around the ribs and sides of the abdomen. Use this stretch if you spend long periods sitting or after an ab workout.

1) Stand with your back straight, chest up, shoulders back, and neck neutral.
2) Raise your left arm straight up overhead.
3) Exhale and reach over the top of your head to the right side, and you should feel a stretch on the left side of your abdomen. Hold this position for 30 seconds.
4) Inhale, release the hold and come back to the center.
5) Switch arms and repeat.

Pelvic Tilt

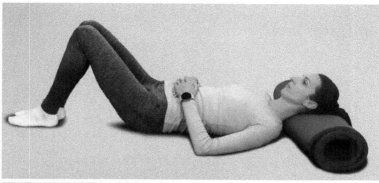

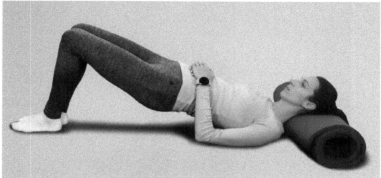

63. A woman performs a pelvic tilt while using a pillow

This stretch will help to strengthen the abs while also relieving tightness in your lower back. The pelvic tilt should be used after leg day, back day, or regularly to improve ab strength.

1) Lie flat on the floor with your knees bent, and your feet comfortably planted flat on the floor.

2) Engage or tighten your abdominals and press your back flat into the floor.

3) Hold this position for 10 seconds; breathe normally.

4) Exhale and release your abs and back. Rest for 15 seconds.

5) Repeat this for 3 sets of three repetitions.

Triceps

Overhead Triceps Stretch

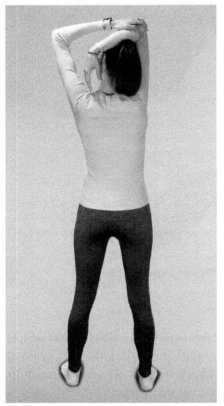

64. A woman performing a triceps stretch

This move will stretch the shoulder and triceps muscles and is a good option for after shoulder, chest, or back day.

1) Sit or stand with your back straight, chest up, shoulders back, and neck neutral.

2) Bring your left arm overhead and reach your forearm behind your head. Your left hand should hang down between your shoulder blades. Keep your bicep close by your ear.

3) Grab your left arm above your bent elbow with your right arm and pull down and towards the right until you feel a stretch. Hold this position for 30 seconds.

4) Switch arms and repeat.

Biceps

Biceps Stretch

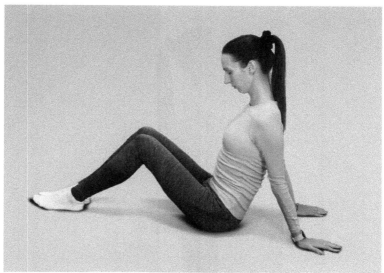

65. A woman performs a seated biceps stretch

This stretch will help stretch out your biceps while opening your chest and shoulders. This stretch is good for relieving upper body tension. Use this move after being sedentary at work or after arms or shoulder workouts.

1) Sit on the floor with your knees bent and feet flat on the ground.

2) Place your palms on the floor with your fingers pointing straight behind the body.

3) Scoot your butt forward slowly until you feel a stretch in your biceps.

4) Hold this position for 30 seconds.

Chest

Chest Stretch

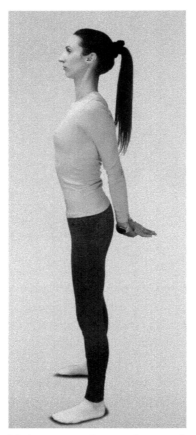

66. A woman performs a chest stretch

This stretch will open up your chest and shoulders. Use this stretch after chest day or when exercising the upper body.

1) Stand with your back straight, chest up, shoulders back, and neck neutral.

2) Reach your extended arms behind your body and interlock your fingers near your buttocks.

3) Keep your shoulder blades back and down and pull your arms out and away from the body until you feel a stretch in your chest. Hold this position for 30 seconds.

4) Exhale and lower your arms back down to release the stretch.

Bent-Arm Wall Stretch

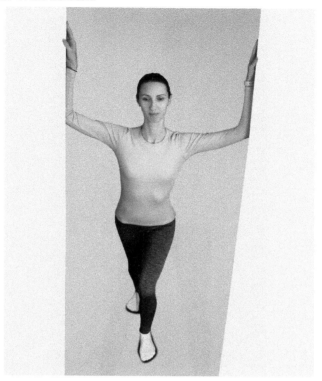

67. A woman stretching in the doorway

This stretch requires a wall or doorway to perform and can be done one arm at a time or with both arms between a doorway. Use this stretch to relieve tension in the chest and help improve flexibility after chest day.

1) Stand up with a straight back and neutral neck in a doorway. Move your feet into a split stance with the left slightly in front and the right behind you.

2) Bring your right arm up to shoulder height with the elbow bent 90 degrees. Place your palm and forearm on the wall. Here your thumb should be slightly higher than your ear.

3) Exhale and press your chest forward into the open space. The arm on the wall will provide resistance and cause you to feel a stretch on that side.

4) Hold this position for 30 seconds.

5) Inhale and pull back out of the stretch.

6) Switch arms and repeat on the other side.

Chest Expansions

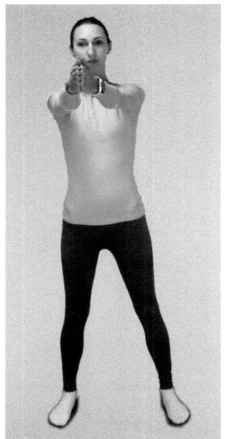

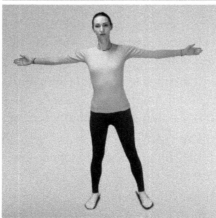

68. A woman performing chest expansions

1) Stand with legs slightly wider than hip-width apart. Keep your back straight and neck neutral.

2) Raise your extended arms up to shoulder height with palms facing each other.

3) Bring your palms close together. Exhale and spread your arms out to your sides, so they are perpendicular to your body and parallel to the floor.

4) Inhale and return arms straight out in front of you, leaving only a small space between palms.

5) Repeat this movement 5 times.

Dumbbell Chest Fly

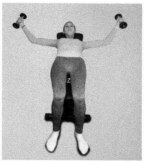

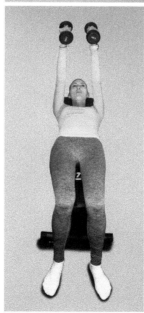

69. A dumbbell chest fly performed on an exercise ball

Use this to help warm up the chest and shoulders before lifting. This movement will provide a stretch across the chest.

1) Grab two lightweight dumbbells. Lie on your back on a flat bench.

2) Extend your arms and dumbbells out to your sides at chest level. Keep a slight bend in the elbow.

3) Exhale and bring your arms together above and in front of your chest, like giving someone a big hug. The dumbbells should come very close to one another.

4) Inhale and slowly return the dumbbells out to your sides.

5) Repeat this movement for 3 sets of 3 repetitions. Rest for 30 seconds between sets.

   Regression: Perform this movement with no weight.

   Progression: Slowly count to 5 as you lower the weight down.

Knee Pushups

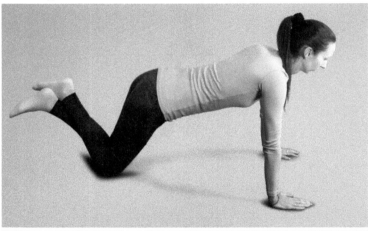

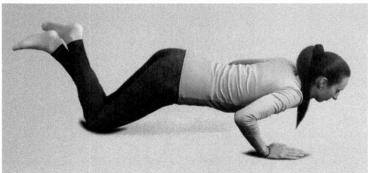

70. A woman performs knee pushups

Use this slightly easier pushup variation to warm up your chest and upper body for push day. This exercise can also be used in place of actual pushups if they are too difficult.

1) Begin prone on the ground with your hands palm-down on either side of your chest. Keep your back straight and neck neutral. Your elbows should be bent and back rather than flaring out to the sides.

2) Bend your knees and cross your lower legs. Your lower legs should be off the ground.

3) Exhale and press up through your palms, and using your chest and triceps, lift your upper body off the ground. Use your knees to support your lower body and keep it planted on the floor. Press up until your arms are almost fully extended, but do not lock out your elbows.

4) Inhale and slowly lower your upper body back down to the floor.

5) For a warmup: Repeat this for movement for 3 sets of 3 reps. Rest for 30 seconds between sets. For a reduced pushup variation, perform this movement for 3 sets of 10 reps, resting 1 minute between sets.

Wrist

Flexion and Extension

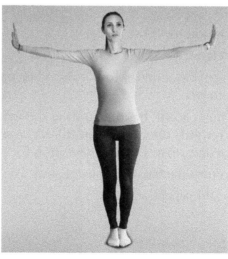

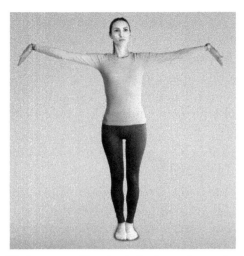

71. A woman with wrists in flexion and extension

This stretch will help loosen up your wrist for greater flexibility. Use this stretch before or after weightlifting or regularly, especially if you type daily.

1) Stand with your back straight, chest up, shoulders back, and neck neutral.

2) Extend one arm straight out in front of you at shoulder height.

3) Use the opposite hand to grab the finger just above the palm.

4) Exhale and pull back on the fingers until you feel a stretch in the wrist.

5) Hold this position for 30 seconds.

6) Inhale and release the hold back to neutral.

7) Keep your arm extended. Move your other hand, so it is now on top of your fingers.

8) Exhale and push down, bending only at the wrist until your fingers are pointed towards the floor. You will feel a stretch on the top of your forearm and wrist. Hold this position for 30 seconds.

9) Inhale and return the wrist back to neutral.

10) Switch arms and repeat.

Wrist Eights

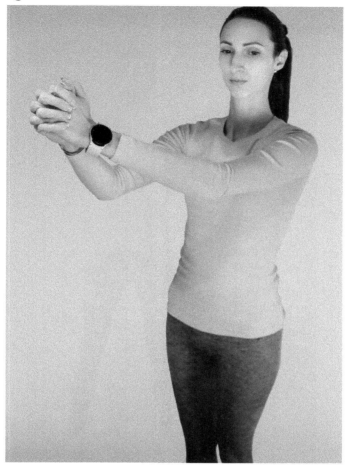

72. Hands interlocked for wrist eights

This movement will help to warm up the wrist joint and loosen tightness in the forearms. This movement should be used regularly or to warm up for exercising.

1) Interlace your fingers in front of your body. Keep your elbows bent at 90 degrees and tucked in by your sides.

2) Rotating your wrists, only move your locked hands in a figure eight motion. Your hands should alternate positions as you move them through the shape.

3) Perform this exercise for 30 seconds.

Shoulders

Cross-Body Stretch

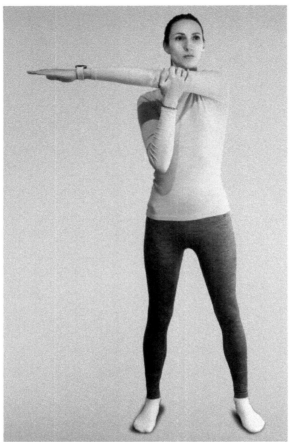

73. A woman performs a cross-body stretch

This stretch will help to release tightness in your upper back and loosen up the shoulders. Use this stretch after a back or shoulder day.

1) Stand with your back straight, chest up, shoulders back, and neck neutral.

2) Grab your left arm around the triceps with your right hand. Pull the arm across your body in front of your chest. Keep your elbows below shoulder height. You should feel a stretch in your shoulder. Hold this position for 30 seconds.

3) Release the stretch and switch arms before repeating.

Shoulder Rolls

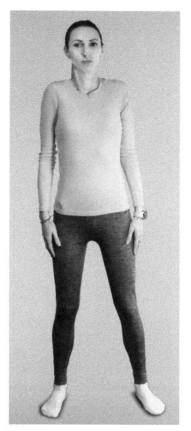

74. A woman performs shoulder rolls

This movement is a good warm-up for your shoulders and will help improve mobility and reset your posture. This move should be used before or after upper body workouts.

1) Stand with your back straight, chest up, shoulders back, and neck neutral. Your arms should hang loosely by your sides.

2) Inhale and shrug your shoulders up towards your ears. Once up, pull your shoulders back and down by squeezing your shoulder blades together. Your elbows should also move back and inward as you perform this motion.

3) Exhale and roll the shoulders forward and back down.

4) Return to the neutral position and repeat.

5) Perform this movement 10 times.

Shoulder Rotation

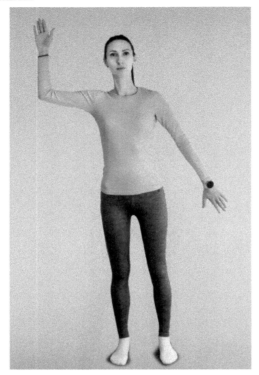

75. A woman performs shoulder rotations

This stretching movement will require a wall to perform and help improve your shoulder mobility. Try this movement before or after an upper body workout or regularly.

1) Stand with your back against the wall and keep your neck neutral.

2) Bend your elbows to 90 degrees and raise them up to shoulder height. Your palms should be facing the floor while you keep the back of your upper arms against the wall.

3) Rotate your right arm in this position up until the back of your hand is flat against the wall. Your thumb should be slightly above ear level.

4) Rotate your left arm downwards while maintaining the same positioning until your palm is flat on the wall. Your thumb should end up at about hip height.

5) Hold this position for 30 seconds.

6) Switch arm positioning and hold again for 30 seconds.

Arm Circles

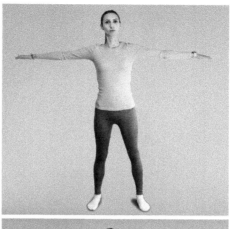

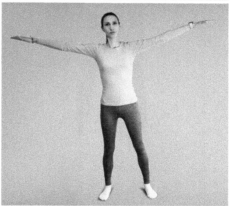

76. A woman performs arm circles

These should be used before most upper body exercises as they help loosen up the arms and shoulders.

1) Stand with a straight back and neutral neck. Keep your chest up. Your feet should be close together.

2) Extend your arms straight out to the sides so they are parallel to the floor at shoulder height and face your palms to the floor.

3) Rotate the arms in forwarding circles. The circles can be small to medium in size.

4) Do this for about 5 complete rotations.

5) Rotate the arms in backward circles for another 5 rotations.

6) Switch your palms so they are facing forward, backward, and toward the ceiling, and repeat the forward and backward rotations.

I, Y, T Stretch

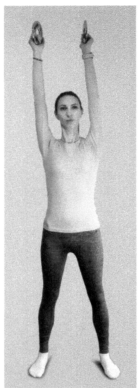

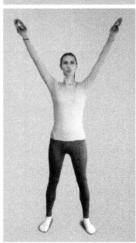

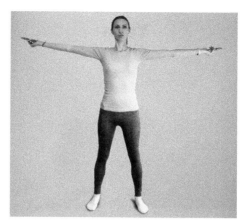

77. A woman performs I, Y, T raises with weights

These should be used before all upper body workouts.

1) Stand with arms about hip-width apart. Keep your back straight, neck neutral, and chest up.

2) Raise your arms so they are straight out in front of you and are extended at shoulder height.

3) Exhale and raise your arms up straight overhead to create an "I" Pause briefly and feel the stretch.

4) Inhale and lower your arms back down to shoulder height.

5) Exhale and raise your extended arms up and out wider than the body to create a "Y" with your arms and body. Pause briefly and feel the stretch.

6) Inhale and return arms to shoulder height.

7) Exhale and spread your extended arms out to the sides at shoulder height. Spread your arms so they only go slightly behind the body at the farthest to create a "T" with your arms and body. Pause briefly and feel the stretch.

8) Inhale and return to your arms to shoulder height in front of you.

9) Repeat this series five times in a row.

Yoga

Child's Pose

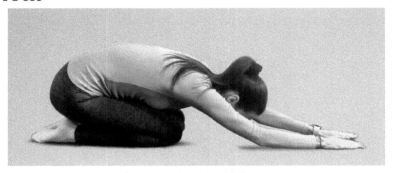

78. An exerciser in a child's pose

This movement is good for the back, glutes, and hips, and it is also helpful for relieving tension and stress.

1) Get on all fours on the floor with your palms flat. Your arms should be slightly in front of you, and the tops of your feet should be against the floor.

2) Exhale and sink back with your hips until you rest your buttocks back on your heels. Your belly will lay on your thighs.

3) When you've sunk back into the pose, breathe deeply and focus on calming the mind and body. Hold this position for 1 minute.

4) Inhale and come up out of the pose.

Sphinx

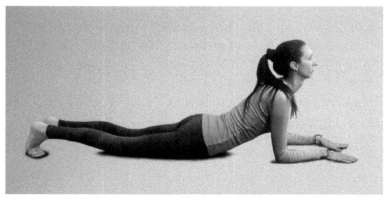

79. A woman performing a sphinx pose

This pose will help to open your back and chest, and it can relieve tension or help with reestablishing posture.

1) Lie prone with your elbows underneath your shoulders and hands flat on the ground out in front of you.

2) Your feet should be slightly apart.

3) Exhale and slowly lift your head and chest. Try to maintain a neutral neck. Your lower body should stay flat on the floor as you press your pelvis down. Lift up until you feel a slight stretch. Hold this position for 30 seconds.

4) Inhale and lower back down.

Pigeon Pose

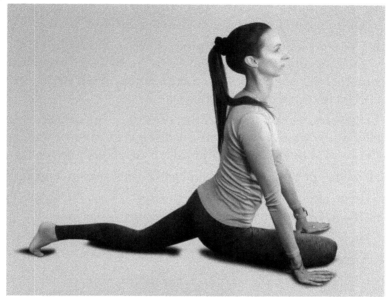

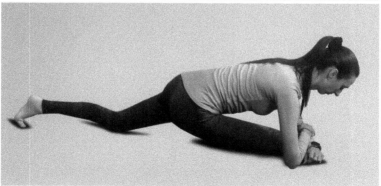

80. A woman performs a pigeon pose

This move will help to stretch out the hips and lower back. This pose especially benefits those who are sedentary for much of the day.

1) Get down on all fours with your hands flat on the floor.

2) Bring your right knee forward and out towards your wrist and lay the outside of it on the floor. The bottom of your right foot should be facing to your left, with your toes pointing forward. Your shin will either be straight in front of you or angled slightly back toward the body. Your right ankle should be somewhere around your left hip.

3) Move your left leg back and straighten it directly behind you. Your thigh and knee should be on the floor.

4) Inhale and lengthen your spine, draw your navel inward toward your spine and open your chest. Use your hands on either side of you to help raise up into this position. Your head should be upright and your neck neutral.

5) Exhale and slowly lower to the floor before you. Your forearms and palms should be flat on the ground in front of you, and your forehead should be down towards or resting on the mat.

6) Hold this position for a 5 count while focusing on your breathing.

7) Exhale and push up with your arms to release the pose. Lift your hips and bring your legs into the all-fours position.

8) Switch legs and repeat.

Eagle Arms

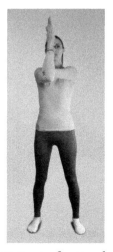

81. A woman performs eagle arms

This movement will help increase flexibility in the wrist and arms.

1) Extend your arms out in front of you.

2) Cross your left arm over and on top of the right.

3) Move your left elbow into the right elbow crook. The backs of your hands will be touching.

4) Move your left arm left and past the right hand. At the same time, move the right arm right. Your palms should end up facing one another.

5) Keep your palms together and left up with your hands. Do not lift your shoulders. Your fingers should be pointing towards the ceiling. Hold this position for 30 seconds.

6) Switch arm and hand positions and repeat.

Downward Facing Dog

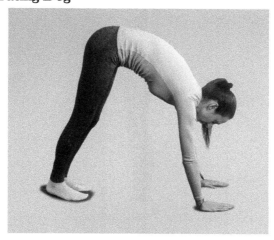

82. A woman in a downward facing dog pose

This movement is used frequently in yoga and often employed to transition from one move to another. It will stretch the hamstrings and calves while building upper body strength.

1) Get down on all fours on the ground with your wrist directly under your shoulders.

2) Curl your toes and push back with your hands to raise your hips up until your legs are straight. Keep your fingers wide for more support, and slightly rotate your arms outward. Your head will be hanging down. Be sure to push your shoulder blades down towards your buttocks.

3) Engage your quadriceps and transfer the weight of your body to them. Rotate your thighs inward and push your tailbone up higher. Try to keep your heels pressed into the floor. Don't move your feet forward to try and lower the heels.

4) Exhale, bend your knees, and lower back down onto all fours.

Mountain Pose

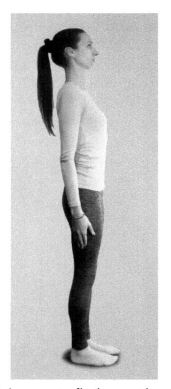

83. A woman standing in mountain pose

This pose is simple but can help relieve stress and improve your posture.

1) Stand with your back straight, chest up, shoulders back, and neck neutral. Your hands should be straight down at your sides, and your feet should be close together and fully planted on the floor.

2) Lengthen your spine, tuck the tailbone, and straighten your legs. Inhale and extend your arms up overhead and then slightly back. This motion should cause a stretch in your upper body.

3) Exhale and gently lower your shoulder blades down and release your arms back down to your sides.

Warrior I

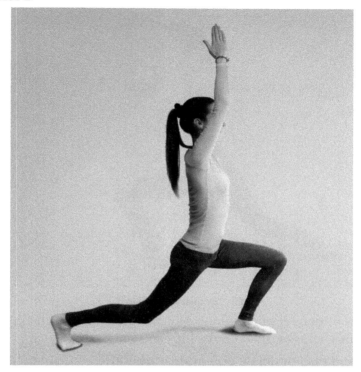

84. A women in warrior I

This pose will build strength in the legs, open up your chest and hips, and awaken your arms.

1) Begin in Mountain Pose with arms raised up and back overhead.

2) Exhale and step your right foot back so you are in a lunge position. Your leg should remain somewhat straight, and your left knee should be over your left ankle.

3) Push up further through your arms and turn your right foot 90 degrees. Your right heel should be perpendicular to the left heel. Check your shoulders to make sure they are pulled back and down. Keep your hips facing forward. Breathe in and out while holding this position for 30 seconds.

4) Inhale, lower your arms, and bring your back foot in and under your body. Return to a neutral stance with arms down by your side.

Warrior II

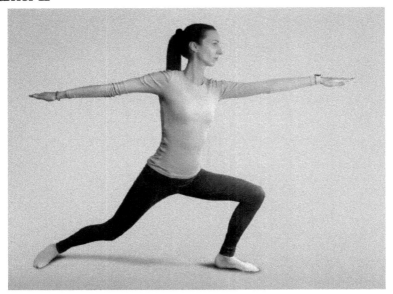

85. A woman in Warrior II

This movement is an add-on to Warrior I. It will turn the pose slightly so that it also helps to open up the hips and hip flexors.

1) Stand in a mountain pose with arms down.

2) Exhale and step your right foot back about four feet into a lunge. Your back heel should remain in line with your front heel.

3) Turn your back heel 90 degrees so your toes point to the side and should be perpendicular to the front foot.

4) Raise your arms extended up to shoulder height. Bring your left arm in front of you and your right arm behind you. Keep your fingers pointing straight out.

5) Bend the left knee so it is directly over the left ankle.

6) Sink down so that your front thigh is parallel to the ground. Look straight out over your front arm. Breathe as you hold this position for 30 seconds.

7) Inhale and slowly lower your arms down to your sides before bringing your back leg into a neutral standing position. Return to mountain pose with arms at your side.

Plank Pose

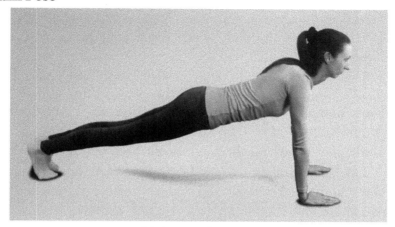

86. A woman in a plank

A plank helps to build strength in the core, arms, and shoulders.

1) Begin on all fours on the floor.

2) Inhale and extend your legs straight out back behind you. Your hands should be directly below your shoulders.

3) Your body should form a straight line almost parallel to the floor. Press up through your hands and push your thighs toward the ceiling. You should feel the weight in your belly as you hold your body up.

4) Breathe as you hold this position for 1 minute.

Bridge Pose

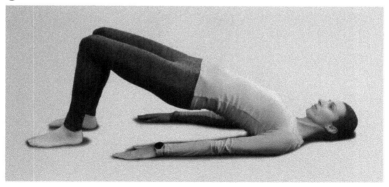

87. A woman in a bridge pose

This move helps to stretch and strengthen the core and lower back.

1) Lie on your back with your knees bent and feet on the floor. Your feet should be hip-width apart. Bring your heels close to your buttocks.

2) Exhale and press up through your feet as you raise your hips up as high as they will go. Lead with the pelvis. Your mid and lower back, buttocks, and legs should be off the floor, and your thighs should be parallel to the floor.

3) Bring your hands together under your back on the floor.

4) Exhale and bring your hands back out to your sides as you return down to the start position.

Tree Pose

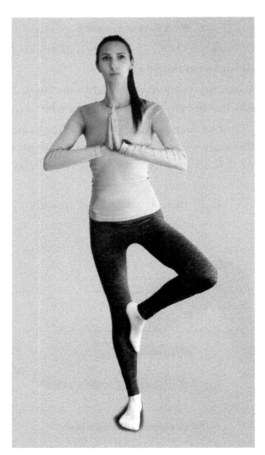

88. A woman in a tree pose

This pose can help you improve your posture and balance.

1) Stand with your back straight, chest up, shoulders back, and neck neutral.

2) Press down through your legs and spread your toes.

3) Exhale and bring your shoulder blades down and back.

4) Place your hands on your hips and raise your left foot up and onto your shin or thigh. Do not put pressure on the knee.

5) Press your left foot and right leg firmly together.

6) Exhale and bring your arms up to prayer pose at chest level before extending them fully overhead. Take 3 breaths in and out.

7) Lower your arms and legs back to the starting position.

8) Switch legs and repeat.

Triangle Pose

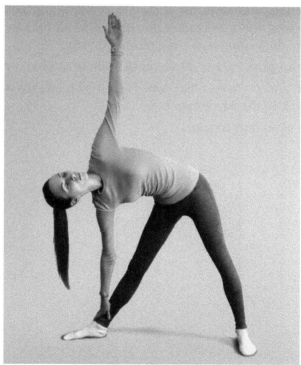

89. A woman in a triangle pose

This movement will awaken the spine and help strengthen thigh muscles. This pose is also a good option for stretching most areas of the body together.

1) Stand in the Mountain pose with arms down.

2) Bring your extended arms out to your sides at shoulder height with your palms facing the ground. Spread your legs out wider than hip-width apart.

3) Turn your left foot outward and your right foot to 90 degrees. Your left and right heel should remain inline, and your legs should remain straight.

4) Exhale and bending from the hip rather than the waist, extend over to the left as far as you can, leading with your right hand. Reach out over the left leg. Hold your right hip firmly in place out to the right to help keep your balance. Press into the ground with your right leg and heel.

5) Bring your left arm down to the floor outside your left calf or rest it on your calf. Your right arm will be pointed straight up toward the ceiling, and both arms should remain straight and extended throughout the movement. Turn your head and look straight up towards the ceiling past your extended arm.

6) Hold this position for 30 seconds while breathing normally.

7) Inhale and press through your back heel to get up out of the pose and back to the Mountain pose.

8) Switch sides and repeat.

Chapter 3: Push: Chest and Triceps

Working the chest, triceps, and shoulders all incorporate "pushing" movements. These exercises involve using your muscles to push objects away from your body or to push your body away from a surface. These exercises are great for building upper body strength, muscle, and power.

When performed regularly, they will increase the muscle in your shoulders and triceps, which help make you look more physically fit. These shirt-filling muscles tend to show nicely when exercised, and the work performed will be noticeable to you and others. Exercising your chest can help firm it up by adding muscle and burning fat.

Exercising the triceps and shoulder will help to keep the shoulder and elbow joints healthy. You use these repeatedly daily, and as you age, keeping them strong and flexible is even more crucial. Putting these muscles and joints under tension and moving them through their full range of motion can help you maintain strength for functional movements. Regularly exercising the shoulder and elbow will reduce your risk of injuring these sensitive areas in everyday activities.

The chest is the primary power source on the front of the body. Keeping the chest strong gives you pushing power that you can apply to getting up off the ground, moving heavy objects, or simply closing a stubborn door. Exercising the chest also incorporates the shoulders and triceps as accessory muscles to help do the work and therefore benefit as well.

Remember to know your limits when exercising the shoulders, chest, and triceps. Listen to your body when it comes to that next rep or using a heavier weight. The goal is to get a workout in without being injured and be able to come back and do it again. If you feel any pain in the neck, back, hips, or any joint you're using, safely cease the exercise as soon as possible. You can always return to it, modify it to an easier variation, or save it for your next push workout.

Chest
Warm-Ups

Chest Expansions

Chest Fly

Knee Pushups

Wrist Eights

Workout

Pushups

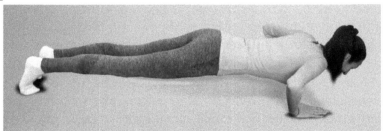

90. A senior doing pushups

1) Begin prone on the ground with your hands palm-down on either side of your chest.

2) Keep your back straight and neck neutral. Your elbows should be bent and back rather than flaring out to the sides.

3) Your legs should be extended straight out with your feet supporting your lower body on the floor.

4) Exhale and press up through your palms, and using your chest and triceps, lift your upper body off the ground.

5) Use your feet to support your lower body and keep it planted on the floor.

6) Press up until your arms are almost fully extended, but do not lock out your elbows.

7) Inhale and slowly lower your upper body back down to the floor.

8) Repeat this for 3 sets of 10 reps, resting 1 minute between sets.

Progression: When lowering yourself back down to the ground, slowly count to 5 before letting yourself all the way down. Or, when pressing up, raise one arm up and tap the opposite shoulder before lowering yourself down.

Bench Press

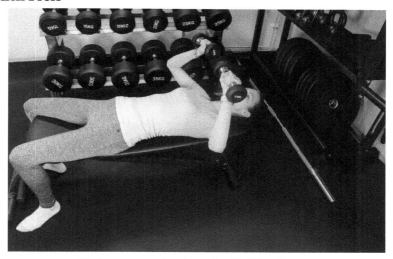

91. A woman performing a dumbbell bench press

In the gym, this can be done on a bench with a barbell or at a Smith Machine with the barbell connected to a slider.

1) Grab a pair of dumbbells and lie on your back on a flat bench. Plant your feet on the floor on either side for support.

2) Hold the dumbbells at your sides slightly above the chest. Keep your wrists in line with your elbows.

3) Exhale and press the dumbbells up, extending your arms using your chest and triceps to provide the pushing force. Squeeze your chest as you press the weight upward.

4) Inhale and lower the weights back down beside your chest. Your elbows should flare down and wide.

5) Repeat this movement for 3 sets of 10 reps with 60 seconds of rest between sets. Increase the weight between sets if desired.

Intermediate progression: Perform the exercise with one dumbbell at a time. Rest the free hand on your chest while you press to feel the muscle engage. Or slowly count to five as you lower the weights down to your sides to increase the time the muscles work.

Incline Bench Press

Before lying on the bench, reach underneath and address the back support. Move it up, so it is at a 45-degree angle from the bench's seat. This adjustment will hit the shoulders differently and target the upper muscles of the chest.

Decline Bench Press

Before lying down to perform the bench press reach underneath and lower the support to its bottom setting. This will put your upper body lower than the seat and force you to press at a unique angle. A decline bench will help target the lower muscles on the chest.

Dumbbell Pullover

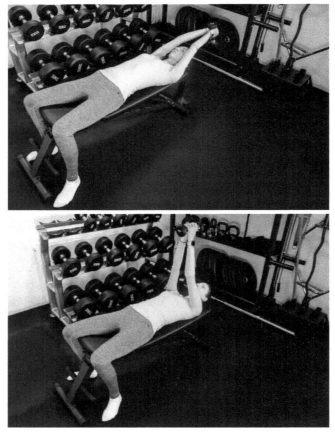

92. A woman performs a dumbbell pullover

1) Grab a dumbbell and lie with your upper back on a flat bench. Your body will be perpendicular to the bench. Keep your lower body straight and in line with your upper body. Your feet should be planted flat on the floor to support the lower body.

2) Keeping a slight bend in your elbow, hold the weight above your forehead.

3) Inhale and lift the weight back and above your head until your feel a stretch in your chest.

4) Exhale, and keeping your arms in the same position, pull the dumbbell up and over your face. The weight should end its movement over your forehead.

5) Repeat this movement for 3 sets of 8 reps. Rest for 60 seconds between sets.

Regression: Use a smaller range of motion when moving the weight back.

Progression: To increase the difficulty, you can increase the weight or repetitions to 10 or 12.

Mid Cable Flys

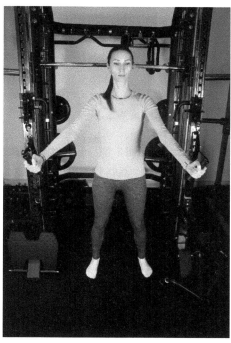

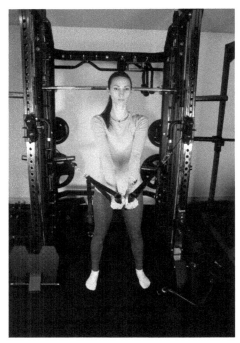
93. A woman performs mid cable flys

These can be performed at a cable machine at home or the gym. The levels of the cable can be adjusted to hit the chest differently. This exercise can also be performed with n anchored resistance band.

1) Adjust the cables on either side of you, so they are at hip height. Grab a handle on each side. Keep a straight back and neck neutral. Lead with your chest.

2) Step forward with your legs staggered. The front leg should be bent, and the back leg should be kept straight. Raise your back leg up onto tiptoes if needed. Keep your arms mostly straight with a slight bend in the elbows.

3) Exhale and pull your arms forward under chest level. Your hands should almost touch.

4) Inhale and slowly let your arms back until they align with your body. Do not let them go too far back.

5) Repeat this movement for 3 sets of 10 reps if done as its own exercise. If used alongside high or low cable flys, perform less.

Low Flys

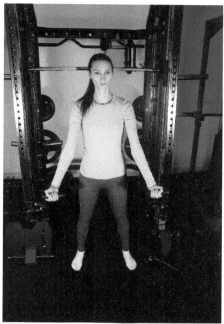

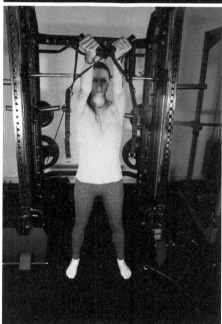

94. A woman performs low cable flys

1) Adjust the cables to be at the lowest setting on each side.

2) Use the same form as the middle flys to get into position. Turn your palms slightly upward, facing in front of you.

3) Exhale and bring your arms up as if you are hugging something round. Your hands should end at the height of the top of your chest.

4) Repeat this movement for 3 sets of 10 reps if done as its own exercise. If used alongside high or middle cable flys perform less.

High Cable Flys

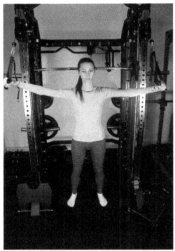

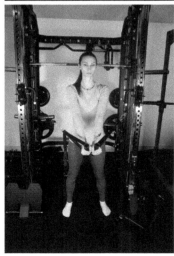

95. A woman performs high cable flys

1) Adjust the cables to be at the highest setting on each side.

2) Grab the handles and get into the same position as the middle flys.

3) When you bring your arms forward, scoop under your chest to engage it, then bring your hands together at chest height to complete the movement.

4) Repeat this movement for 3 sets of 10 reps if done as its own exercise. If used alongside low or middle cable flys perform less.

Regression: Perform this movement with little to no weight to stretch and prime the muscles usually used.

Progression: To increase the difficulty, slowly count 5 as you release your arms back from out in front of you to increase the time the muscles are engaged under the weight.

Triceps

Warmup

Arm Circles

Overhead triceps stretch

I, Y, T Stretch

Dips

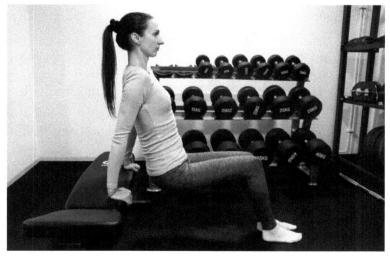

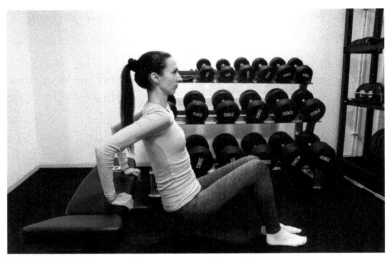
96. A woman performs dips

1) Use a bench or a secure chair with a hard flat surface.

2) Stand in front of the bench with your back to it.

3) Lower yourself down and put your hands slightly wider than your shoulder width apart on the bench. Palms will be on the bench, and the tops of your fingers will be facing the same way you are.

4) Bend the knees to a 90-degree angle and place your feet on the floor out in front of you. Keep your head up and back straight. Your butt should be at the level of the bench but in front of it rather than sitting on it.

5) Inhale and bending only at the elbows; lower your body down. Your elbow should get to almost a 90-degree angle, and your buttocks and lower body will dip toward the ground right in front of the bench.

6) Exhale and squeeze your triceps and press yourself back up until your arms are almost fully extended.

7) Repeat this for 3 sets of 10 reps, resting for 30 seconds to a minute between sets.

Regression: Only go down halfway or perform the movement seated in a chair holding the arms as you dip.

Progression: Move your feet out further until your knees are at about a 45-degree angle. Or extend your legs out straight and place your heels only on the ground in front of you.

Close Grip Bench

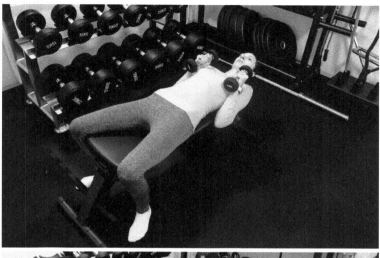

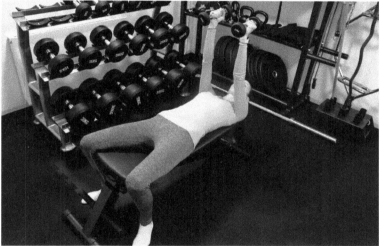

97. A woman performs a close grip incline bench press

This exercise can also be performed with a barbell or on a Smith Machine. When using these two options, keep your hands about shoulder-width apart on the bar. Don't go too narrow.

1) Grab two dumbbells and lie on your back on a flat bench. Plant your feet securely on the floor.

2) Begin with the dumbbells just above your body, slightly below your chest. Keep your elbows close to your sides.

3) Exhale and squeeze your triceps to press the dumbbells up and out in front of your body. Your elbows should almost be straight at the top, but do not lock your elbows out.

4) Inhale and slowly lower the dumbbells down to the starting position.

5) Repeat this movement for 3 sets of 10 reps. Rest for 60 seconds between sets.

Regression: Perform the movement with a lighter weight

Progression: After pressing the weight up, slowly count down to 5 as your lower the dumbbells back down to the start.

Triceps Pushups

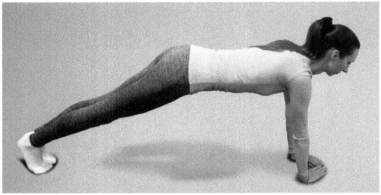

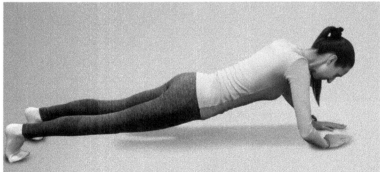

98. A woman performs triceps pushups

1) Get onto your hands and knees on the floor and allow your lower legs to rest on the ground straight behind you.

2) Place your hands close together in a diamond shape on the ground between chest and shoulder height. Keep your back straight.

3) Inhale and slowly lower your upper body down to the ground by bending at the elbows only. Do not flare the elbows out to the side. They should bend straight back.

4) Exhale and squeeze your triceps to press your upper body up until your arms are extended.

5) Repeat this for 3 sets of 8 reps and rest for 60 seconds between sets.

Progression: Increase the reps to 10-12 for an increased challenge. Or lift your knees off the ground, so you are in a plank position. Only your feet and hands will be in contact with the ground.

Overhead Triceps Extension

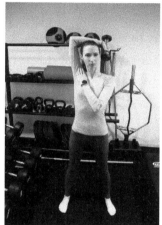

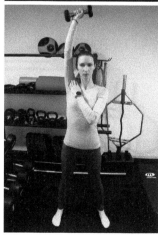

99. A woman performs an overhead triceps extension

This exercise can be performed with a dumbbell, resistance band, or cable machine. When using a cable machine or resistance band, the tension is kept tight and on the muscle throughout the movement.

1) Grab a single dumbbell. Stand with your feet slightly wider than hip-width apart. Keep a slight arch in your back. Keep your neck neutral.

2) Hold the single dumbbell behind your head by grabbing the end of the handle where it connects to the weight. Your wrists should remain straight in line with your forearms, and your elbows should be in front of you and bent to 90 degrees. Engage your core to help support the weight being lifted over your head.

3) Exhale, and using the triceps, press the weight up until it is directly overhead. Keep your wrists straight throughout. The weight should end directly overhead with your arms extended above you.

4) Inhale and lower the weight back down behind your head.

5) Repeat this movement for 3 sets of 10 reps. Rest for 30 seconds between sets.

Regression: Perform the movement holding a water bottle or rolled-up socks.

Progression: When lowering the weight back down, slowly count to 5 to increase the time the muscles support the weight.

Triceps Pushdown

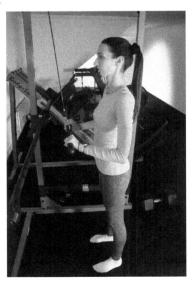

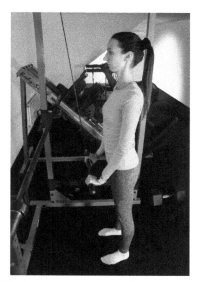
100. A woman performs a triceps extension

This exercise can be performed with a cable machine or anchored resistance band.

1) Securely anchor your resistance band to a high point. Stand with feet hip-width apart. Keep your back straight and neck neutral. Don't let your shoulders roll forward. Use a short bar handle or hold the resistance band handles with hands closer than shoulder width.

2) Pull the weight down so the handle is at about chest height. Your elbows will be bent to almost 45 degrees and by your sides. Do not flare them out to the sides. Engage your core to keep from allowing the pull of bands to move you.

3) Exhale and straighten the arms at the elbow as you push the handles down and to the top of your thighs. Squeeze your triceps and keep your wrists straight.

4) Inhale and return the handle back to the top of the movement.

5) Repeat this movement for 3 sets of 12 reps. Rest for 60 seconds between sets.

Regression: reduce the weight.

Progression: After pressing the weight down, slowly count to 5 as you release the weight back up to the starting position.

Dumbbell Kickback

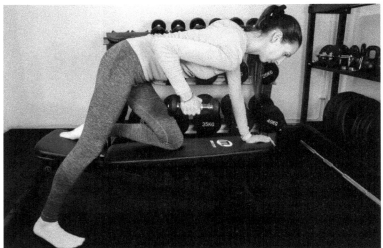

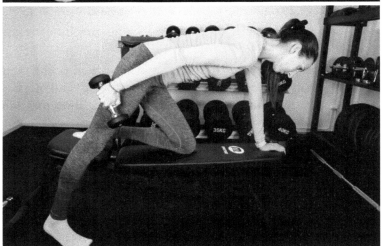

101. A woman performs a triceps kickback

1) Grab a single dumbbell. Usually, lighter is better for this isolated movement. Place one bent knee on a flat bench. The knee on the bench will be on the opposite side of the dumbbell, and the other leg should be on the floor beside the bench, slightly bent. Bend over, so your back is almost parallel to the ground but keep a slight arch.

2) Place your free hand on the bench to help support your body. Keep a neutral neck. Lift the elbow holding the dumbbell up, so it is slightly higher than your body. Your upper arm will be parallel

to the ground, and your elbow will begin bent at 90 degrees.

3) Exhale and use your triceps to straighten your arm and kick the dumbbell straight back.

4) Inhale and lower the weight back down, so your elbow is at a 90-degree angle.

5) Perform this exercise for 3 sets of 8 reps. Rest for 30- 60 seconds between sets.

6) Switch sides and repeat using the other arm.

Regression: Perform the movement while holding rolled-up socks.

Progression: To make this exercise harder, increase your reps.

Shoulders

Warmups

Arm Circles

I, Y, T

Shoulder Rolls

Shoulder Press

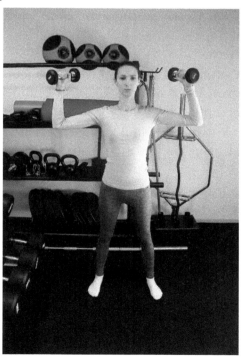

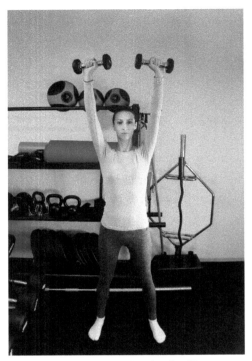
102. A woman performing the shoulder press

This movement can be done with a barbell or a resistance band anchored under your feet.

1) Grab a pair of dumbbells. Stand with your feet slightly wider than hip-width apart. Keep your back straight and neck neutral. Engage your core to support the weight you'll be handling overhead.

2) Raise your arms up to shoulder height. Bend your elbows to 90 degrees and keep your wrist straight. Your palms will be facing forward.

3) Exhale and press the weight straight up overhead. The weights should end up above your head. Your arms will come closer together at the top of the movement but don't straighten them.

4) Inhale and lower the arms back down to the starting position.

5) Repeat this movement for 3 sets of 10 reps. Rest for 1 minute between sets.

Regression: Perform the movement holding water bottles or rolled-up socks.

Progression: Instead of using two dumbbells, only use one. Be sure to keep your body straight and don't move it to compensate for the weight. Or after lifting the weight, overhead count to 5 as you slowly lower the weight back down to the start.

Bent Lateral Raise

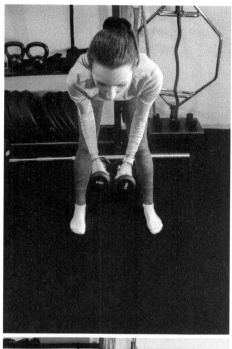

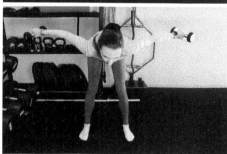

103. A woman performing a bent lateral raise

This exercise can be performed using dumbbells, cable machines, or resistance bands. When using the cable or band, begin the movement with a single cable or anchored band pulled tight on the opposite side from where you will be pulling. Perform the movement one arm at a time.

1) Grab a pair of lighter dumbbells and stand with feet hip-width apart. Bend your upper body about 45 degrees. Keep your neck neutral, and don't round the back.

2) Hold the weights straight down in front of your chest. Keep a slight bend in your elbows.

3) Lead with your elbows. Exhale and spread your arms out to your side until your upper arms are in line with your body.

4) Inhale and lower the weights back down to the starting position.

5) Perform this movement for 3 sets of 10 reps. Rest for 1 minute between sets.

Regression: Perform the movement with rolled-up socks or no weight

Progression: After the weight has been lifted out to your sides, slowly count to 5 as you lower the weights back down.

When using cables: Securely attach a cable or band low on your left side. Get into the same starting position above. Grab the cable with your right hand and pull it across your body to get it into the starting position. Lift the weight using one arm at a time. Switch arms and repeat.

Front Raise

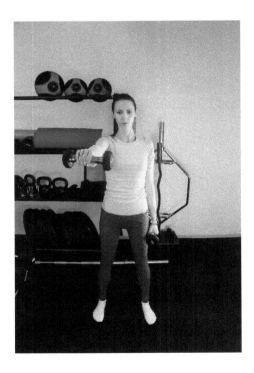

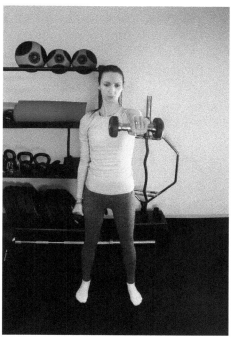

104. A woman performs a dumbbell front raise

This exercise can be performed with dumbbells, cables, or bands attached low and behind you.

1) Grab your dumbbells. Stand with feet hip-width apart. Keep your back straight and neck neutral.

2) Start with the dumbbells in front of your thighs. Keep a slight bend in your elbow and wrists straight. Keep your arms about shoulder-width apart. Engage your core to help offset the weight.

3) Exhale and raise your arms up and out in front of you to shoulder height.

4) Inhale and slowly lower the weight back down to your thighs.

5) Repeat this movement for 3 sets of 10 reps. Rest for 60 seconds between sets.

Regression: Perform the exercise with water bottles or rolled-up socks

Progression: To increase the difficulty, after raising the weight up, slowly lower it back down as you count to 5. Or this exercise can also be done with a single dumbbell. Be sure not to use your body to offset the weight. Instead, engage your core and control the weight.

When using cables: Attach the cable to the lowest part of the machine or band to a low anchor. Garb the handle and stand in front of the machine with your back to it. The cable handle should begin by the outside of the thigh on the arm holding the handle.

Lateral Raise

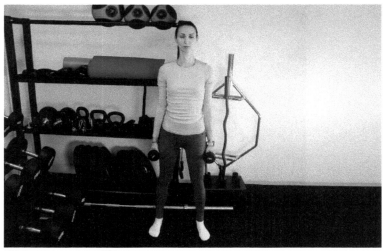

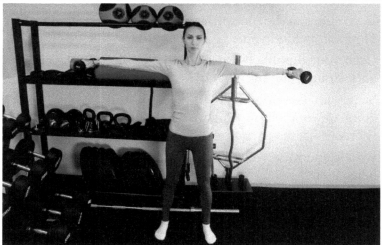

105. A woman performs dumbbell lateral raises

This exercise can be performed using a dumbbell, cable machine, or anchored resistance band.

1) Grab a dumbbell. Stand with feet hip-width apart. Keeping your back straight and neck neutral. Engage your core.

2) Begin with the dumbbell on the outside of the thigh of the hand holding it. Keep your wrist straight but put a slight bend in the elbow.

3) Exhale and raise your arm up and out to the side. You do not need to lift it all the way to shoulder height. You should feel your shoulder working as you raise the weight.

4) Inhale and lower the weight back down to your thigh.

5) Repeat this for 3 sets of 8 reps. Rets for 60 seconds between sets.

Regression: Perform the exercise while holding rolled-up pair of socks.

Progression: To make this exercise more challenging, increase the time it takes to lower the weight back down to your sides by counting to 5, if possible, as you lower it.

When using a cable or band:

1. Anchor the cable to a low point.

2. Stand sideways to the anchor point of the cable.

3. Grab the handle with the hand on the side opposite the cable and pull it across the body. The cable handle should begin just in front of the thigh, further away from the cable anchor.

Face Pulls

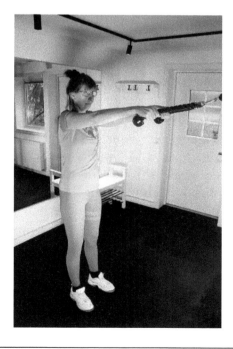

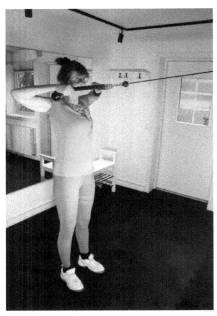
106. A woman performs standing face pulls

1) Sit or stand with your cable attached at a height above your face. You will need two handles for this, *with one anchored point.* If using a cable machine, the double rope attachment should be used if possible. If standing, keep your knees slightly bent and feet wider than hip-width apart.

2) Keep your back straight and neck neutral. Engage your core to help compensate for the pull of the weight. Begin with your arms at shoulder height with elbows at 90 degrees in front of you, holding the cables. Keep your wrists straight.

3) Exhale, and leading with your hands, pull the cables back until your upper arms form a "T" with your body. Elbows will remain at a 90-degree angle throughout the movement. Your hands should end slightly behind your head. Open your chest and squeeze your shoulder blades together when as you pull.

4) Inhale and let your arms return to out in front of you.

5) Perform 2 sets of 10 reps. Rest for 60 seconds between sets.

Regression: Use as light a band as possible

Progression: After pulling the cable back so your arms are in line with your body, keep your arms in the same position but raise them straight up overhead while keeping the tension in your shoulders, back, and cable.

Chapter 4: Pull: Back and Biceps

Ever try opening the fridge and have trouble? It's likely because the door is stubborn, but it could also be because you've lost some pulling power. Either way, it's frustrating, yet when the door is stuck, having good pulling power can make opening it possible. Another scenario where pulling power would be life-changing is if you were to fall and end up on the floor. Being able to grab onto a door handle or the railing of a staircase and pull yourself up is vital.

Pulling power comes from the back and biceps muscles on the front of the upper arm. Keeping these muscles strong will allow you to pull things closer to you without falling over and allow you to pull yourself closer to a fixed object. The biceps are smaller than the back, so they serve as accessories and support the greater pulling power of the back.

The back acts as the anchor for the body and is the power base for your limbs. As you use your back in most functional movements, such as squatting, keeping it fit can make them more manageable. The back also supports the shoulder and shoulder blades, invaluable areas we constantly use that are susceptible to injury. Remember, the back muscles support the spine too, which constantly endures our body weight and movement.

Exercising your back can also help to improve posture and reduce pain. If sitting hunched over at your desk is the cause of poor posture, then exercising your back is the cure. Keeping your back muscles strong and flexible can help to hold your body in proper alignment. This can help you look and feel better as your joints sit as they are intended to.

In addition, exercising your back and biceps can be fun as you get to pull weight around. Below you'll find plenty of functional pulling exercises for the back and biceps. Take advantage of them and start with lightweight, so you enjoy the full engagement of the muscle as you exercise your pull muscles.

Be sure to listen to your body as you exercise. If you feel any pain in your back, neck, chest, or another area, cease exercising immediately. When a weight feels too heavy, either lower it or return to it later. Remember, the goal is to reduce pain, increase functional strength, improve posture, and come back and exercise tomorrow.

Warm-Up

Wrist Eights

Cat Cow

I, Y, T Stretch

Biceps Stretch

IYT Raises

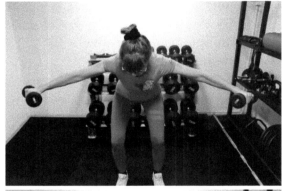
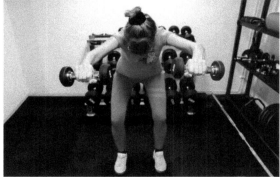

107. A woman performs I and T raises

This exercise can either be done standing up and bent at the hips or lying prone on an exercise bench or stability ball.

1) Grab a pair of light dumbbells and bend over at the waist by pushing your hips back. The dumbbells should be hanging down in front of you.

2) Allow your arms to extend and face your palms inward.

3) Exhale and raise your arms straight up before you until they are parallel to the ground. Your elbows should be by your ears, and you will form an "I" with your arms and upper torso.

4) Inhale and lower them back down to the starting position.

5) Exhale and raise your arms up but spread them out into a "V" formation until they are parallel to the ground, so they form a "Y" with your torso.

6) Inhale and lower them back down to the starting position.

7) Turn your palms so they are facing each other. Exhale and raise your arms up and out to the sides until they are parallel to the ground. Your palms should be facing the ground, forming a "T" formation with your arms and upper torso.

8) Inhale and lower your arms back to the start.

9) Repeat this process for 3 sets of 8 repetitions. Rest for 60 seconds between sets.

Regression: To make this exercise easier, you can perform the movement with no weight or use water bottles.

Progression: To increase the difficulty, count slowly to 5 as your lower the weights each time.

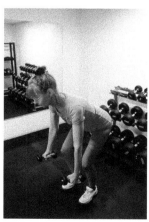

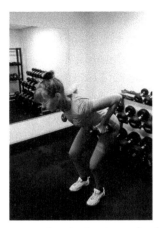
108. A woman performing bent-over dumbbell rows

This exercise can alternately be performed using an exercise band anchored underneath your feet, a barbell, or a substitute weighted item such as a backpack.

1) Grab a pair of dumbbells and stand with your feet shoulder-width apart. Keep a neutral neck.

2) Bend over by pushing the hips back. Keep your back mostly straight with a slight arch. Your upper body should be at about a 45-degree angle. Allow the weights to hang down in front of you with your elbows extended and palms facing each other.

3) Exhale bend at the elbows, and, leading with your elbows, pull the weight up towards either side of your ribcage. Your arms should stay tucked in close to your body, and the move should end with your elbows slightly behind your back.

4) Inhale and lower the weight back down to the starting position.

5) Repeat this movement for 3 sets of 10 reps with 60 seconds of rest in between.

Regression: Instead of weights, try using water bottles.

Progression: Try lifting and lowering the dumbbells one at a time; this will help with improving stability. Or count to 5 as you slowly lower the weight back down.

Seated Cable Row

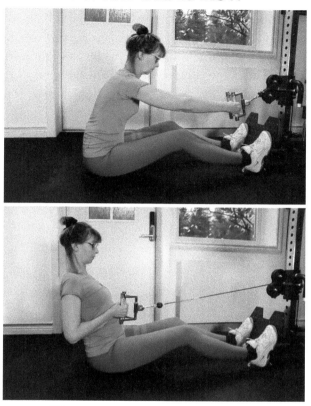

109. A woman performing seated cable rows

This movement can be performed using a cable machine or anchored resistance band.

1) Adjust the cable, so it is at about chest height when seated in front of it. Grab a V bar, rope, short bar, or other attachment. Sit down with a straight back and neutral neck. Plant your feet flat in the foot supports if using a cable machine.

2) Begin the movement with your arms extended with a slight bend in the elbow. Engage your core to brace for the pull of the weight.

3) Exhale and, leading with your elbows, pull the handle straight in toward the bottom of your chest. Bend your elbows and lead with them as you pull. Your elbows should end up behind your body.

4) Inhale, slowly extend your arms, and allow the weight to return to the starting point.

5) Repeat this movement for 3 sets of 10 repetitions. Rest for 60 seconds between sets.

Regression: Reduce the weight of this exercise if it feels too heavy.

Progression: Slowly count to 5 when releasing the weight back to the starting position. Or use a single handle and less weight and perform the movement with one arm at a time to further engage your core.

Straight Arm Pulldown

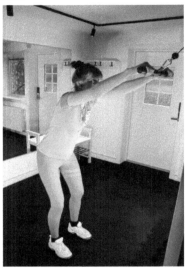

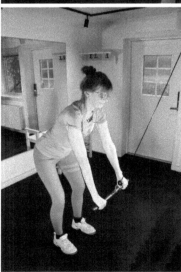

110. A woman performs straight arm pulldowns

This can be performed with a cable machine or high anchored resistance band such as the top of a door.

1) Adjust the cable to the highest point on the machine. Use a straight bar, if possible, or turn resistance handles so that your palms are facing the floor.

2) Step back about two feet from the anchor point. Keep your feet close together and arms extended. Bend slightly at the waist and keep a slight arch in your back. Begin with your arms extended out at a 45-degree angle.

3) Engage your core. Exhale, and keeping the arms straight, pull the bar down and in toward the tops of your thighs by squeezing your lat muscles located on your back below the armpit.

4) Inhale and slowly release the cable back to the starting position.

5) Perform this movement for 3 sets of 8 reps with 30-60 seconds of rest between sets.

Regression: Reduce the weight.

Progression: Slowly count to 5 as you return the weight to the starting position.

Lat Pulldown

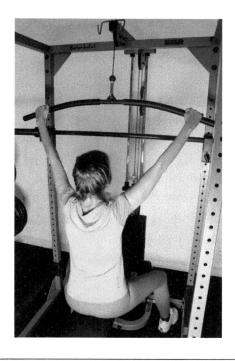

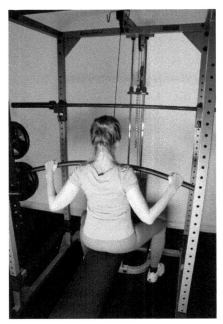

111. A woman performs a lat pulldown

This exercise requires a cable machine or a high anchor point and resistance band.

1) Attach the long lat bar bent on the ends. Sit with a straight back and secure your legs with the thigh bar if using a machine. If using bands, sit on the floor or chair.

2) Grab the bar just outside shoulder width with palms facing forward. Lean back slightly. Engage your core. Begin with your arms extended and above you by pulling the cable tight and beginning to bear the weight with your biceps and back.

3) Exhale and pull the bar down and toward your chest. The bar should end at about mid-chest, and your elbows bent and pointed toward the floor somewhat behind your back.

4) Inhale and slowly release the bar back up to the starting position.

5) Repeat this movement for 3 sets of 10 reps with 60 seconds in between sets.

Regression: Reduce the weight.

Progression: Slowly count to 5 as you release the weight back to the starting position. Or use a single arm handle and only work using one arm at a time.

Pull-up

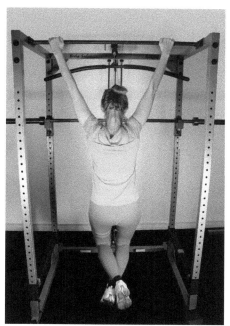

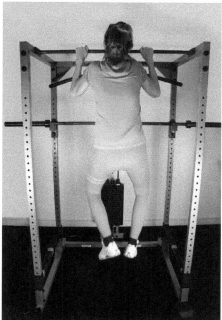

112. A woman performs a pull-up

This exercise will require a pull-up bar on a collapsible pull-up frame anchored in a doorway or part of a designated pull-up tower. This exercise uses the same movement as a lat pulldown. However, it is more difficult as it requires raising your entire body weight.

1) Reach up and grab the bar slightly wider than shoulder-width apart. Your arms should be fully extended as your grip the bar.

2) Exhale, engage your back and biceps, and bend your elbows as you pull yourself up toward the bar. Lead with your chin and try to pull your chest up to bar height.

3) Inhale and lower yourself back down to the starting position.

4) Repeat this movement for 3 sets of 10 reps. Rest for 60 seconds between sets.

Regression: Use an assisted pull-up machine or purchase an assisted pull-up band.

Progression: Switch your grip so your palms face you to further engage the biceps. Or try to hold yourself at the top of the pull-up before lowering yourself down. Or weight can also be added by wearing a packed backpack or weight vest.

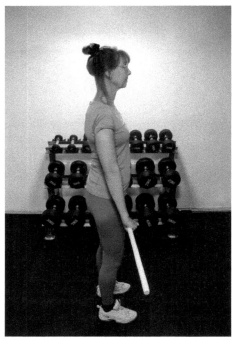

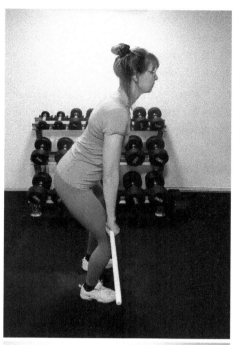

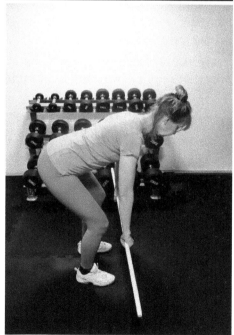

113. A woman demonstrates a Romanian deadlift

This is a compound movement and one of the most beneficial in weightlifting. It uses muscles on the back, plus the glutes, hamstrings, and arms. This exercise can be used as a leg exercise as well. The movement can be done with a barbell, resistance band, or dumbbells.

1) Grab a pair of dumbbells and hold them shoulder width apart with your palms facing you. Stand with legs about hip-width apart. Keep your back mostly straight with a slight arch and your neck neutral.

2) Bend the knees slightly and engage your core and back. Keep your arms extended throughout the movement. The weight should begin in front of your thighs.

3) Inhale and hinge at the hips to lower the weight to your shins. If you cannot go that low, go as far as possible.

4) Exhale and push forward with your hips while pulling up and back with your back to return to the starting upright position. Squeeze your glutes as you pull up.

5) Repeat this movement for 3 sets of 8, resting for 60 seconds between sets.

Regression: Reduce the weight and practice hinging at the hip and engaging the core and back during the motion.

Progression: Increase the weight and reduce the reps to build greater power. Or slowly lower the weight down with a 5 count after pulling it up.

Superman

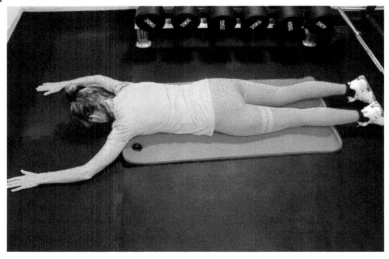

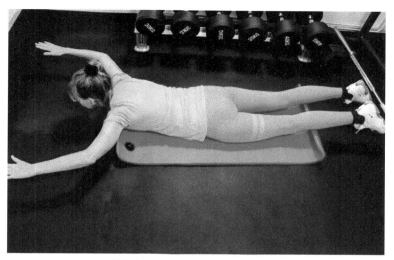

114. A woman performs Supermans

1) Begin lying prone on the ground with arms extended straight overhead, palms facing down, and the tops of your feet on the floor.

2) Keep a neutral neck as your look at the floor directly below your face.

3) Inhale and raise your arms and legs up off the ground without bending the knees or elbows. Your head and most of your chest should be off the ground as well. Hold this position for 30 seconds

4) Exhale and slowly lower your body to the starting position.

5) Repeat this 3 times, resting for 30 seconds in between.

Regression: Reduce the duration of your hold to 15 seconds

Progression: Hold the position for 45 seconds. Or slowly raise and lower into the hold 3 times before engaging for the 30-second hold.

Biceps

Biceps Curl

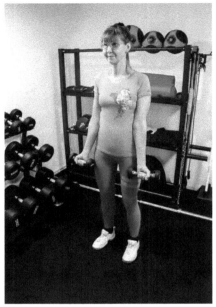

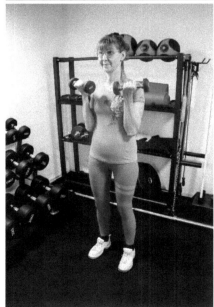

115. A woman performs standing dumbbell biceps curls

This exercise can alternatively be done with a barbell, curl bar, resistance bands, or substitute weights such as water bottles.

1) Grab a pair of dumbbells with palms facing forward and stand with legs hip-width part. Keep a straight back and neutral neck.

2) Begin with the weight in front of your thighs.

3) Exhale and bend the elbow past a 90-degree angle as you squeeze the biceps and pull the weight up. Don't swing the weight. The weight should end up around shoulder height, and your upper arms should stay close to the sides of the body.

4) Inhale and lower the weight back down to the starting position.

5) Repeat this for 3 sets of 10 reps with 60 seconds of rest between sets.

Regression: Raise the weight only up to a 90-degree angle in the elbow. Or hold the weight at a 90-degree angle in the elbow for up to 30 seconds at a time without curling the weight up. Then release it back down and rest for 60 seconds.

Progression: Raise the weight one arm at a time, left, then right, before lifting them both together for each rep.

Hammer Curl: For a variation on the movement, turn the handles or dumbbells so palms are facing each other, and the weight looks like a hammer as it raises and lowers.

Isometric Biceps Hold

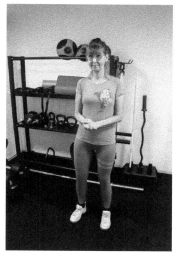

116. Exercisers perform an isometric biceps hold

1) Stand with arms about hip-width apart. Keep your back straight, shoulders back, and neck neutral.
2) Extend your arms out in front with a wider than 90-degree bend in the elbow.
3) Press your palms together.
4) Inhale and press your palms together with force without letting your arms move. Try to bear the weight of the press in the biceps. Continue to press for 30 seconds, if possible, before releasing.
5) Exhale and release the press.
6) Repeat 3 times with 30 seconds rest in between.

Chapter 5: Legs: Quads, Hamstrings, and Calves

The legs are your movers; when they aren't strong enough to work, everything can be harder. As a senior, you've likely been using your legs daily for the last 60 years, and that's a lot of wear and tear. There may likely be pain, weakness, or imbalances you wish weren't holding you back. Luckily you can exercise them and build stability, flexibility, and strength.

With strong legs, getting up from your chair and walking across the room is not an issue. The legs are significant to keep fit as once they become too weak to hold you up and move you, your ability to move and stay active begins to fade. The legs are crucial to keeping your independence. Strong legs can help prevent unnecessary falls or injuries, which can be devastating to a senior.

Exercising the legs also helps to keep your bones strong. Maintaining bone health is essential for seniors because they can lose mass over time and become fragile. Exercise can serve as a treatment to help strengthen your joints and bones as a protective measure against a severe injury.

The exercises listed below are all commonly used in weightlifting, bodybuilding, and strength building for athletes. While they can be loaded with heavy weight, they serve just as much purpose when performed regularly with light weight. Use these exercises to build a strong base that can hold up and move your body when you want it to.

If you feel any weakness or pain in your knees, back, hips, or other joints, stop exercising immediately! These exercises aim to get you strong and confident enough to move freely. Listen to your body and modify an exercise if it feels too difficult. Make sure to get your leg day in and perform these movements at least once a week.

Warm-ups

Wall Stretch

Knee to Chest

Leg swings

Lateral leg swings

Wall Sit

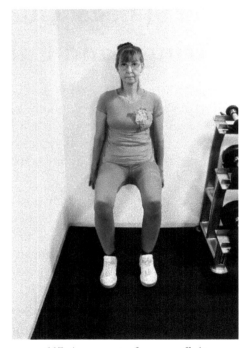

117. A woman performs a wall sit

1) Lean against a wall with your back. Scoot your butt down until your legs are at a 90-degree angle and your thighs are parallel to the floor. Your feet will be out and away from the wall, and your legs should be about shoulder-width apart.

2) Get comfortable in this position with your back and top of your butt pressed flat against the wall and feet planted securely. Keep your hands flat on the wall with palms facing down.

3) Once securely in place, hold this position for 30 seconds if possible. Stand up to complete the movement.

4) Repeat this movement 3 times, resting for 30 seconds between holds.

Squat

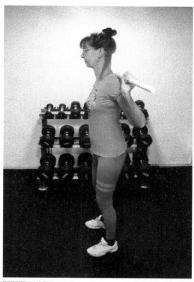

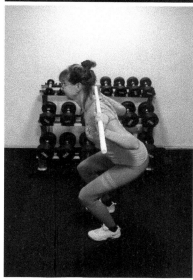

118. A woman performs a barbell squat

This exercise can be performed with a barbell on your back, dumbbells on your shoulders, or a dumbbell held in front of your chest.

1) Grab a barbell and place it on your upper back. Hold the bar just outside shoulder width with palms facing forward. Stand with your feet wider than hip-width apart and toes pointed forward or slightly outward. Keep a straight back, chest up, and neutral neck.

2) Inhale, engage your core, push your hips back and bend your knees. Lower down as if sitting back into a chair. The knee should push out over the foot. Don't let it drift inward. Lower down as if sitting back into a chair. Try to get down so that your knees are at 90 degrees.

3) Exhale and press up through your feet as your push your hips forward to stand back up to the starting position.

4) Perform this movement for 3 sets of 10 reps with 60 secs of rest between sets.

Regression: Perform the movement with no weight, and for further support, hold onto the back of a chair in front of you. Or sit back onto a chair or bench for support at the bottom

Progression: Performing this movement with weight may be the progression. Or pause at the bottom of the squat before coming back up.

Deadlift

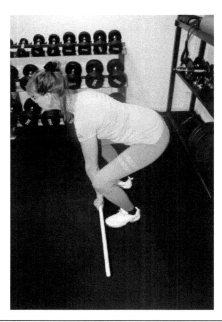

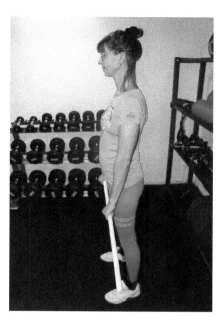

119. A woman performs a barbell deadlift

This movement is like the Romanian Deadlift, but the weight will start on the floor rather than up at the thighs and focus more on the legs and glutes. For this exercise, it will likely be easier to start with a barbell or a similar object like kettlebells with elevated handles you can pick up off the floor with two hands.

1) Stand about hip-width apart in front of the barbell. Your shins should be about touching the bar. Grab the bar about shoulder width with palms facing down. Your hips should be back, and your knees about 90 degrees. Squeeze the bar tightly.

2) Keep your ankles under your knees, your back straight, and your neck neutral. Don't hunch over; your chest should be pointing up at the end of the movement.

3) Exhale, press your feet into the floor and push your hips forward as your pull the bar straight up in front of your body. Engage your hamstrings by slightly pulling your knees back.

4) Continue the movement until you stand up straight with your hips and knees fully extended. The bar should end in front of your thighs.

5) Inhale and push your hips back as you lower the bar back down right in front of your body.

6) Repeat this movement for 3 sets of 8 reps with 60 seconds of rest in between sets.

Regression: Reduce the weight and practice focusing on the movement and improving your flexibility.

Progression: Increase reps or slowly count to 5 as you lower the weight back down.

Floor Bridge

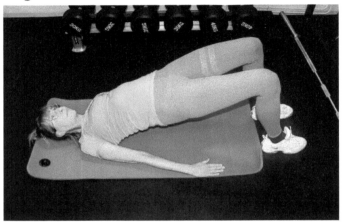

120. A woman performs a floor bridge

1) Lie on your back on the floor with your knees bent to 90 degrees and feet flat. Your legs should be hip-width apart. Place your arms on the floor to your sides. Draw in your abs and keep your back straight throughout

2) Secure your feet and squeeze your glutes as you press up into a bridge. Your butt and lower back should be off the floor and in a straight line with your upper torso.

3) Pause briefly and then slowly lower back down into the starting position.

4) Repeat this for 3 sets of 10 reps and rest for 30 seconds between sets.

Regression: Instead of performing repetitions, squeeze the glutes and raise them up as high as you can into the bridge and hold the position for 10 seconds.

Progression: Extend one leg straight out at the knee at the top of the movement. Lower back down and extend the opposite leg on the next rep.

Lunge

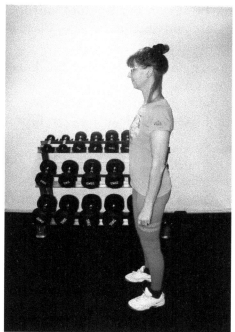

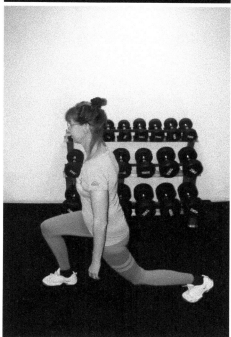

121. A woman performs lunges

1) Stand with the left foot about 2 feet in front of the right. Your back foot will be up on the forefoot and toes. Keep your back straight, chest up, and shoulders back. Place your hands on your hips or up overhead for balance.

2) Inhale and lower down by bending the knees. Your back knee should end up a few inches from the floor, and your front thigh should be parallel to the floor. Distribute your weight evenly between your legs. Don't lean too far forward, and keep your knees straight

3) Exhale and push up through your feet to return to the starting position.

Regression: Don't go all the way to the floor; instead, only drop halfway from the starting position. Or hold onto the back of a chair for support throughout the movement.

Progression: Add light dumbbells in each hand, held straight down by your sides.

Calf Raise

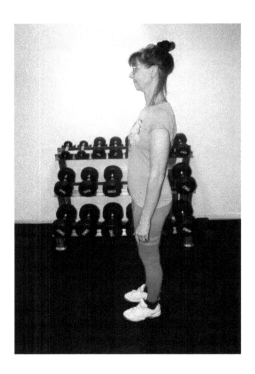

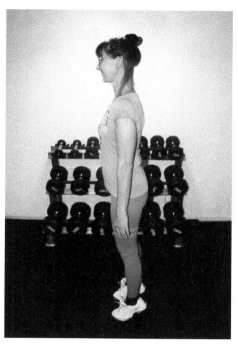

122. A woman performs standing calf raises

1) Stand with your feet shoulder-width apart. Keep your back straight, shoulders back, and neck neutral.

2) Engage the core. Inhale and press up through your forefoot as you raise your heels.

3) Pause at the top when you're as high up on your toes as you can go.

4) Exhale and lower your heels back down.

5) Repeat this movement for 3 sets of 10 reps. Rest for 30-60 seconds between sets.

Regression: Hold onto the back of a chair for support.

Progression: Hold dumbbells in your hands by your sides as you perform the movement.

Chapter 6: Cardio and Core

Cardio isn't precisely a strength training exercise. It can build muscle in the legs, glutes, and core, but it isn't specifically used for this. Cardio is like a supplement to strength training and a crucial aspect of overall health.

Cardio helps to improve your energy and capacity for activity. Regularly participating in cardio exercise increases your ability to exercise for longer without tiring or running out of breath. Not only does this make exercising more manageable, but it translates into functional activities in everyday life. Instead of getting winded walking upstairs, you can keep walking to your destination when your cardio is strong.

Cardio refers to the cardiovascular system, the heart, and blood vessels. They control the flow of oxygen and nutrients throughout the body, which keeps the body feeling good and functioning correctly. Sitting in one place for long periods without moving doesn't feel great, especially when you get up. Cardio is the opposite of this.

Performing cardio regularly will help protect your heart health. Keeping your heart pumping helps to ward off disease and helps ensure that you can keep moving. Cardio also helps keep your joints loose as you use them regularly to move around during exercise.

Lastly, cardio helps you to burn calories and can improve mood and sleep. Your body is expending energy when you perform cardio, such as dancing. This expenditure burns the calories you put in when you eat, and if you burn more than you put in, you can lose weight. When you're done dancing, you will likely feel a boost of energy from getting the blood flowing and raising your heart rate. After this effect wears off, you should feel calmer, and eventually, this can help with sleep habits.

The core is one of those areas you don't think of in the practical sense. When you imagine a strong core, it is probably a bunch of rippling muscles clearly visible and seemingly unattainable. The truth is that a core will look this way because of low body fat, but it doesn't necessarily make the core stronger than one without visible muscles.

The core helps us move. It's involved in turning, bending, and getting up and down. The reason to keep your core strong is so you can move without hurting or hesitation. The core is the middle part of your body opposite your back. Like the back, it is connected to many movements and connects the lower body with the upper. As it serves as the center of the body, it is also responsible for keeping us balanced. Therefore, a strong core helps to prevent falls and reduce the risk of injury.

A strong core can also help to keep the back strong – as they are both parts of the core and provide balance for one another. By exercising the core, you are helping to improve back health and reduce back pain which is common in older adults.

When performing these exercises, be sure to listen to your body. Cardio does exert the heart, so beware of any chest pain. Low-intensity cardio has as many benefits as pushing yourself in an intense session. Cardio is overall healthy, but if it makes you feel unwell, cease the activity and reevaluate.

While core exercises primarily involve body weight, they could strain a body part that may be weaker than you expected. Use regressions, slowly build up to more challenging exercises, and stop performing a movement if you experience pain.

Warm-ups

Abdominal Twist

Side Stretch

Cat-Cow

Plank

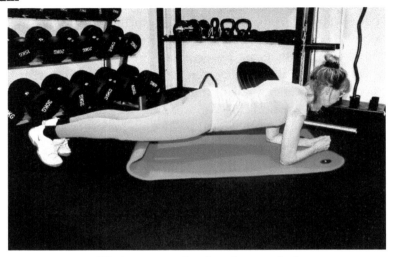

123. A woman performing a forearm plank

1) Start prone on the floor. Your forearms should be on the ground with your thumbs facing the ceiling.

2) Engage your core and push up onto your feet so that only your forearms and feet are in contact with the floor. Your shoulders should be directly above your elbows, and your back should be straight.

3) Hold this position for 10 seconds.

4) Lower yourself back down to the floor.

5) Repeat this hold 3-5 times with 20 seconds of rest in between.

Regression: Instead of extending your legs and using your feet, use your knees as the lower support along with your forearms.

Progression: Raise up onto your hands instead of forearms keeping your elbows fully extended. Or from the forearm position, alternate reaching one arm out in front of you and tap the floor before returning it to the hold.

Arm-Leg Raise

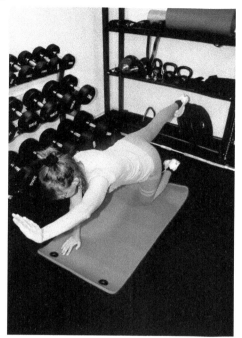

124. A senior performs arm-leg raises

1) Get down on the floor on all fours. Keep your back straight and neck neutral.

2) Extend your right leg straight out behind you to align with your torso. At the same time, extend your left arm straight out in front of you to align with your torso. Your arm and leg, and torso should all be parallel to the floor.

3) Hold this position for 10 seconds

4) Lower down to the starting position. Repeat with the opposite arm and leg.

5) Perform this hold 10 times on each side.

Regression: Only raise your limbs one at a time instead of simultaneously.

Progression: Hold the position for 20 seconds for each rep.

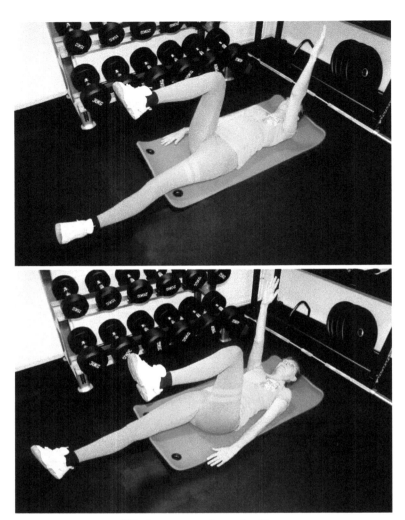

125. A woman performs dead bugs

Dead Bugs

1) Lie on your back. Extend your arms straight up into the air at shoulder height.

2) Raise your legs up off the ground bending the hip and knee to 90 degrees so that the knee is directly over the hip.

3) Inhale and slowly lower your left arm back, so your hand comes close to the ground above your head. At the same time, lower your right leg, so the foot comes close to touching the ground below you.

4) Exhale and raise your arm and leg back up to the starting position.

5) Repeat with the opposite arm and leg.

6) Perform this movement 10 times with each pair of arms and legs.

Regression: Only lower and raise your arms or legs, not both simultaneously.

Progression: Fully extend your legs at the knee through the movement.

Side Bends

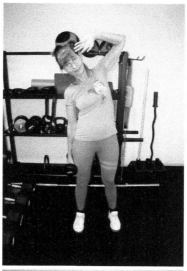

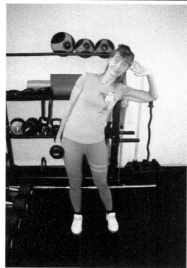

126. A woman performs side bends while holding a dumbbell

1) Stand up with legs hip-width apart. Keep your back straight, chest up, and neck neutral.

2) Place your right arm behind your head with your elbow pointing to the side and your left arm pointing straight down your side by your hip.

3) Engage your core. Crunch your left side while extending your right to lower your left hand further down your side toward the ground. The movement should be small, but your hand should go up and down your side.

4) Use your core to pull your body back to the upright position in the center.

5) Switch arms and sides and repeat.

6) Perform this movement for 3 sets of eight on each side.

Regression: Perform fewer repetitions of the movement.

Progression: Hold a dumbbell in each hand extended down by your side.

Wood Chops

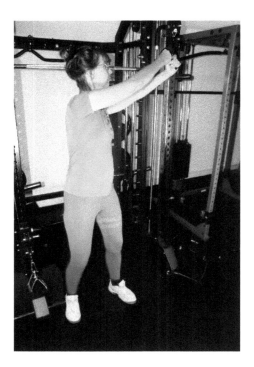

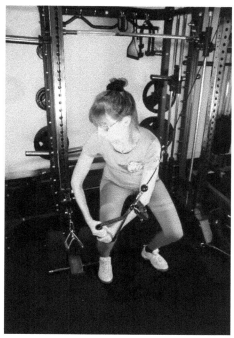
127. A woman performs wood chops using a cable machine

1) Stand with feet shoulder-width apart. Keep your back straight and chest up.

2) Hold your hands clasped in front of you with a slight elbow bend.

3) Engage your core. Inhale and lower your arms down to the outside of your left thigh. Follow the movement of your hand with your head.

4) Exhale and raise your arms up and across the body to above the right shoulder. Our left elbow should end up by the left side of your face.

5) Switch sides and repeat.

6) Perform ten repetitions on each side

Regression: Only raise the arms up to shoulder height.

Progression: Hold a small weight in your hands. Or include a bend in the knees as you lower the weights down. When extending back up, turn the foot that's opposite the way you are raising inward and lift its heel.

Warm-ups

Leg Swings

Lateral Leg Swings

Wall Stretch

Knee to Chest

Dance

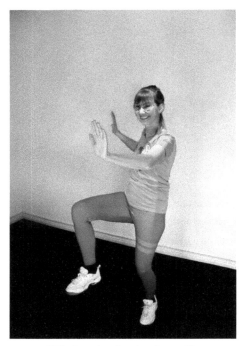

128. A senior dancing for cardio

1) Find an open area in the house with a non-slip surface or wear shoes with an appropriate grip on the tile floor.

2) Put on some upbeat music

3) Check the time and begin to dance. Be sure to incorporate your whole body and move your arms, legs, and hips.

4) Continue moving for 30 minutes max if possible.

Regression: Reduce the duration you are dancing.

March In Place

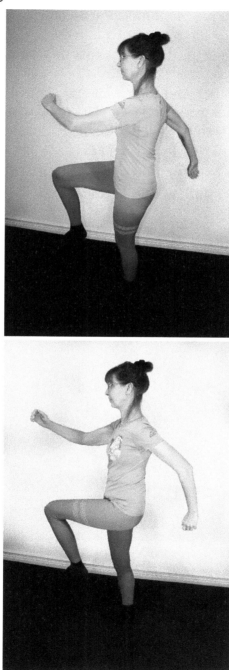

129. A woman marching in place

1) Find a small open area in the house, preferably near the television or where you can play music. Put on an engaging show or upbeat music.

2) Check the time on the clock or set the alarm before you begin. Stand with feet slightly apart.

3) Swing arms back and forth while raising and lowering each leg. Bend the knee as you raise it and try to bring your thigh parallel to the floor on each repetition.

4) Try to keep moving for 15 minutes.

Regression: Only use your arms or legs instead of moving both.

Progression: Hold small weights in your hands.

Walk

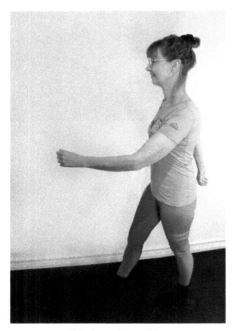

130. A senior walking

This exercise can be done inside on a treadmill if you have one.

1) Plan out a safe place to walk in your neighborhood so that you can estimate the distance or time it will take.

2) Go for a 30-minute walk.

Regression: Reduce the duration to 10 minutes.

Progression: Carry a pair of small weights.

Jog

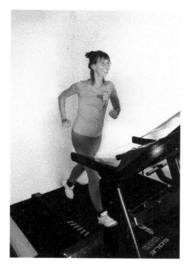

131. A senior jogging

1) Plan out a safe place to jog in your neighborhood so that you can estimate the distance or time it will take.

2) Go for a 15-minute jog keeping a slightly challenging pace.

Regression: Go for a 5-minute jog or slow down to a fast walk.

Progression: Increase the jog duration.

Bike

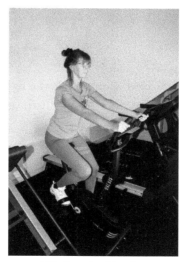

132. A senior bicycling

This exercise can be performed on a stationary bike if possible.

1) Check your bike, including the tires, seat, and brakes, to ensure it is ready to ride. Put on a safety helmet.

2) Plan out a 30-minute bike ride.

3) Ride your bike at a leisurely pace.

Regression: Go for a 10-minute bike ride.

Progression: During your bike ride, attempt to pick up the pace for 2-3 30-second bursts.

Punches & Kicks

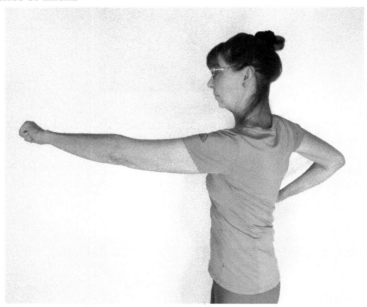

133. An older woman punches for cardio

1) Find an open area in the house with non-slip floors or wear appropriate non-slip shoes.

2) Put on upbeat music or the television. Check the clock before you begin or set the alarm.

3) Stand with knees hip-width apart. Keep facing forward throughout the movement with a straight back and chest up.

4) Sidestep out to your left side, keeping your leg straight. At the same time, punch out to your left with your left arm.

5) Kick forward with your left leg while punching forward with your left arm.

6) Kick behind you with your left leg while reaching back and punching straight back behind you with your left arm. Your elbow should be pointing back behind, and your fist pointing toward the floor as you punch.

7) Switch sides and repeat the whole process.

8) Continue this for 15 minutes if possible.

Regression: Hold onto a chair for support while performing the movements.

Progression: Increase duration to 30 minutes.

Chapter 7: Diet and Why it is Crucial

One of the keys to successful results from exercising doesn't have to do with working out. When you exercise, you are expending energy. The energy comes from burning calories, and those calories must come from somewhere. If you haven't eaten anything, they will come from the body breaking down stored fat or muscle and using that to power you through your workout. Otherwise, whatever you eat for fuel is what the body will use as energy during exercise.

Similarly, after you work out, your body needs refueling to recover from the work you just did. The food you eat after exercising will be used by the body to refill the calories burned and repair and build up the muscle you just worked. Putting in the right foods helps the body function properly and makes this process easier. At the same time, eating healthy and balanced meals should make you feel better regardless of exercise.

Just like choosing premium gas for the car, which food you use as fuel matters. As mentioned before, exercise is difficult for everyone but can be especially tough for seniors. The difficulty level only goes up if you aren't putting good food in for your body to work with. You want to eat balanced meals with various vitamins and nutrients along with a balance of the three major macronutrients.

Everything you eat falls under protein, carbohydrates, or fat. Protein helps to build muscle and is made up of foods like chicken, beef, eggs, almonds, and cottage cheese. Carbohydrates help to provide and replenish energy and can also prevent the body from using any protein or muscle as energy. Carbohydrates include foods with sugars and fiber, such as bananas, rice, bread, potatoes, and oats. Fats help the body produce the energy and hormones needed to build muscle and absorb much-needed nutrients. Foods high in fat include olive oil, avocados, coconut oil, cheese, and some fish.

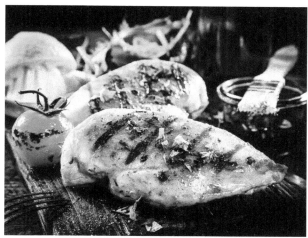

134. Grilled chicken breasts

Protein

Balancing the diet and making sure good sources of all of these are consumed are essential to meeting health goals, especially when exercising. Many consider protein the leader of the three when it comes to exercise. Protein contains the building blocks for muscles; without it, the exercise would not build or strengthen muscles. Seniors lose much of their muscle mass, so eating this protein is extra crucial to help maintain the muscle and strength you have.

High protein is recommended at every meal when working out to get the most out of your nutrition and your workout efforts. The percentage of a general adult's diet that should be protein is between 10%-35%, while carbohydrates should be 45%-65%, and fats should be 20%-35%. It is recommended, though, that seniors get closer to 50% of their daily calories from protein as their bodies may not be able to use what they put in as well.

It's not always easy to get adequate amounts of protein in. Many everyday dishes and snacks such as pasta, pancakes, bread, and fries contain little to no protein. While it is only a portion of what you should be eating, it's probably most important to be sure to get enough when exercising. Protein shakes are a common supplement used by exercisers for just that reason. They are usually a powder mixed with water or pre-bottled and contain 20 grams of protein or more and little else. These shakes are an easy way to get in extra protein without any added carbohydrates or fats to help improve exercise goals. While these shakes can help, it is best to be sure to include protein as a part of every meal or snack to spread it out throughout the day and help increase the chances of hitting your 50%.

Putting good food in also helps to reduce the chances of injury. Eating what your body needs helps it function how it needs to with exercising. By letting your diet slip and not eating enough or overeating junk, you could go into a workout weaker than expected. This weakness may take you by surprise and either result in a sidelining injury, shortened workout, or discouragement when it comes to the next workout. It's tough enough to get a good workout in and then come back again for the next one without dealing with any feelings of fatigue or weakness from a poor diet.

Your food, too, will help you recover better. After your workout, the next part of your work begins with choosing your meals carefully until the next workout. Eating protein helps strengthen your muscles; consuming healthy carbohydrates provides your body energy to keep going, and by eating fats, you allow your body to process the workout and food you put in correctly. A poor diet could lead to aches and pains as your body struggles to recover or fatigue from not putting enough of the good stuff in.

Types of Macronutrients

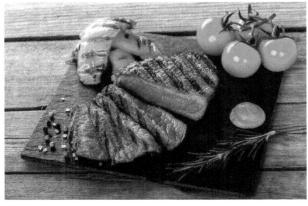

135. Lean steak

When it comes to protein, the leanest or purest is the best. Chicken and turkey, especially white meat, are two of the best standalone protein options. Lean steak and Mahi are two alternatives that are also healthy and beneficial. Egg whites are also commonly used in muscle building for breakfast as they contain valuable protein without the added fat and cholesterol from the yolk of the egg. Any protein helps, though, and it's best to choose what you enjoy so that it is not a chore to add it to your meals and eat it regularly.

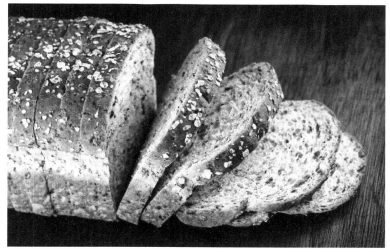

136. Whole grain bread

Carbohydrates can be broken up into two main categories: slow-digesting and fast-digesting. As mentioned, early carbohydrates are energy. Fast-digesting carbohydrates are broken down by the body, making that energy available quickly. Slow-digesting contains fiber which takes the body time to process, slowing down the release of the energy for use. While fast-digesting is good for workouts as it will give you a boost to get through the workout, they aren't good all the time. Once the body burns through those carbs, there will be a drop-off in energy and likely a craving for more. This drop could lead to fatigue and snacking if not accompanied by protein or slow digesting carbs. Slow-digesting carbs can help release slow, sustained energy that can help keep you feeling full longer. This slower release can help prevent snacking or facing constant highs and lows.

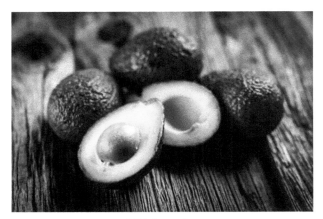

137. Avocados

Fats can also be divided into two main categories. Bad fats are called trans-fat or saturated fat and contribute to risks for many diseases. These fats are usually in delicious treats and sweets such as fried foods, packaged snacks, ice cream, and margarine. They can increase bad cholesterol, lower good cholesterol, and cause inflammation leading to stroke, heart disease, and diabetes. Healthy fats are called monounsaturated and polyunsaturated and can be found in avocadoes, nuts, olives, seeds, and fish. These fats help promote heart health by reducing bad cholesterol and inflammation.

Choose the right mix of these macronutrients to improve your overall health. While they will improve your exercise results, they can also just keep you feeling your best regularly. Remember that you control your independence, and how you feel and ultimately eat properly can play a significant role in both.

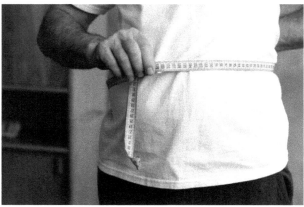

138. A man measures their waist

Weight Loss

While it can be challenging to drop weight as a senior, it is still achievable. Losing weight can be a good way to boost your overall health and help extend your independence. Weight loss may seem like a mystery, but it's just a matter of understanding the way it works.

To lose weight, you must burn more calories than you eat. That is the secret to weight loss. Even if you don't follow a strenuous exercise plan, you can still lose weight by following this simple equation. It comes down to a matter of choosing the right foods, eating the right amount of them, and staying active. By doing this, your body will naturally lose weight that you can keep off. Pay attention to what you are eating and ensure it is filled with nutrients, balance, and foods that will keep you full. Eating high protein and high fiber can help improve your chances of weight loss, and healthy fats can help keep you feeling balanced as you do it.

Your body should only be hungry until you are full, so eating healthy foods will fill you up with good. This should reduce your chances of snacking or eating excess that your body won't use for energy. Once you have your diet down, the next step is staying active. Activity will burn off calories first, targeting the healthy food you are eating and then your body fat. Check the mirror and scale both frequently and notice what works. Use these check-ins to gauge your progress and enjoy your results.

Losing weight provides benefits other than tightening up your body and reducing your pant size. Losing weight means the weight your bones and joints carry is lessened. This relief can reduce pain and help keep you going without injury for longer. This ability is crucial to staying active, which, as you know, is the most important thing as a senior. Losing weight can also help improve your mood, reduce your risk of heart disease, lower your blood pressure, and improve your sleep. These benefits equate to a better overall quality of life and a reduced chance of facing chronic disease.

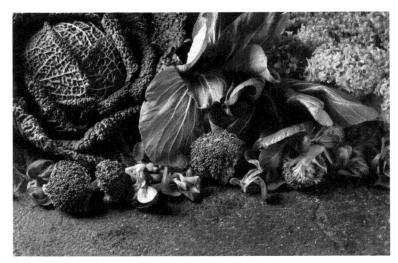
139. A collection of leafy greens

Diabetes

Diabetes is a common condition across the world. It relates to the body's ability to use insulin or glucose, the sugar that comes from carbohydrates. Those with prediabetes or diabetes usually must be very strict with their diet when it comes to carbohydrate consumption. If carbs aren't appropriately managed, symptoms can flare up, and the condition can worsen.

The best thing you can do to manage a diabetes diet is to plan every plate with protein, grains, and healthy fruits and veggies. Whole grains should be slow-digesting options like sweet potatoes, quinoa, or brown rice. For fruits and veggies, focus on getting a good variety of nutrients and plenty of fiber. These options should include leafy greens, broccoli, carrots, squash, brussels sprouts, arugula, lettuce, berries, citrus, and tomatoes. This combination should help leave you feeling full, boost energy, and help with digestion without spiking your sugar levels and triggering unwanted symptoms.

Osteoporosis

Osteoporosis is a bone condition common in older adults. It increases the spaces inside of bones and causes them to become thinner and weaker. This weakness can lead to breaks and cracks that may prevent seniors from being active.

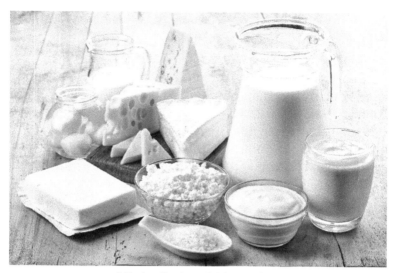
140. A collection of dairy products

To help combat osteoporosis, seniors should eat foods that help boost bone health. The two most essential ingredients are calcium and vitamin D, followed by vitamin K, zinc, magnesium, and protein. Foods to include in your diet are milk, cheese, yogurt, oranges, leafy greens, salmon, eggs, nuts, broccoli, cauliflower, and cabbage.

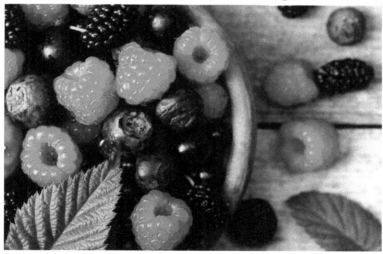
141. A bowl of berries

Kidney Diet

The kidneys help to remove fluid and wastes from your body. They work hard to filter the blood and keep the fluid and electrolytes in the body balanced. Without their constant work, the body would quickly cease to function. Kidneys can wear down over time, but some dietary choices can help.

The primary way to keep the kidneys working is by eating healthy options and restricting certain nutrients. Sodium, potassium, phosphorus, and protein intake must be monitored so the kidneys are not overwhelmed. While these nutrients are needed for the body to function, the kidneys will have trouble filtering and removing them if they are present in excess. Healthy recommended options include berries, fatty fish, egg whites, cruciferous vegetables, garlic, and buckwheat.

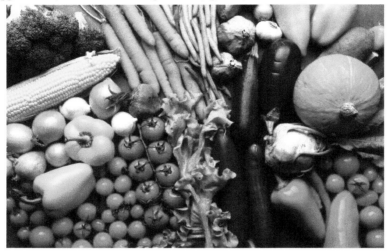

142. A variety of vegetables

Liver Health

The liver, like the kidneys, also helps process the blood flowing through the body. It removes toxins and processes nutrients so the body can use them properly. A healthy liver diet aims to get the proper nutrients and balance without overwhelming the liver.

The liver is responsible for breaking down and using proteins that the body needs, but this can take a toll. Reducing protein intake to adequate levels should be the top priority for those with liver health. Avoid high sodium foods and shellfish. Be sure to fill the lack of protein with higher amounts of good carbohydrates and moderate healthy fats. This diet should include fruits, vegetables, oats, grains, fiber, beans, and dairy.

Recipes

Grilled Chicken and Potatoes

This is a basic dinner or lunch recipe with high protein, healthy fat, and carbohydrates. The chicken can be used for a sandwich on wheat or whole grain bread instead of being served with a full meal.

Ingredients

- 2 Chicken breasts or 6 tenderloins
- 1 lb. Whole potatoes or chopped frozen potatoes, or you can substitute with sweet potatoes
- 1 lb. Brussels sprouts- fresh, bagged, or frozen, or you can substitute with asparagus or broccoli
- 4 tablespoons olive oil
- 1 teaspoon black pepper
- 4 cloves garlic

1) Marinate chicken with a low-sodium seasoning or sauce for a few hours or overnight. Seasonings can include flavors such as barbecue sauce, lemon pepper, spicy, or garlic and herb. Preheat the grill to medium-high heat. Cook the chicken on the grill until the interior temperature is just under 160 and let sit for 5 minutes before eating or serving.

2) Cut off the ends of the Brussels sprouts and remove the yellowish outer leaves. Mix with olive oil, garlic, and pepper and put them on a baking sheet. Preheat the oven to 400 degrees and roast the sprouts for 35 minutes.

3) Cut the potatoes into quarters and mix in a bowl with olive oil, pepper, and garlic. Place the potatoes on a sheet pan. Roast for 45 minutes until browned. Flip the potatoes halfway to ensure they are cooked through.

Baked Salmon and Rice

This is a light and refreshing high-protein and high-healthy fat meal. This dish can be used for dinner or lunch. The salmon can also be covered with a salsa or a pineapple/mango mixture instead of the marinade.

Serves 2

Ingredients

- 2 Salmon fillets
- Olive oil (to marinate)
- ½ teaspoon paprika
- 2 cloves minced garlic
- Pepper (to taste)
- 2 tablespoons lemon juice
- ½ teaspoon onion powder
- 1 lb. or 1 large bunch of asparagus
- 2 teaspoons olive oil
- Red pepper to taste
- 1 cup long-grain brown rice or 1 bag instant brown rice
- 1 tablespoon Sriracha
- Lime juice to taste

1) Preheat the oven to 400 degrees. Cover the salmon in olive oil, paprika, pepper, lemon juice, onion powder, and garlic

2) Place on a baking sheet and bake for at least 12 minutes until the salmon is cooked through. It should be a translucent pink but not completely translucent when done.

3) Remove the woody or white ends that easily snap off the bottom of the asparagus stalk. Cover the asparagus in olive oil, and then add red pepper flakes to taste. Preheat the oven to 425 degrees. Spread asparagus evenly on a sheet pan and place in the oven for 9 minutes for thin or up to 15 minutes for thicker.

4) Cook the bag of instant brown rice in boiling water per instructions. For long-grain brown rice, first, rinse the rice under running water. Add rice and water to a medium saucepan. Cover and bring to a boil, and then set a timer for 30 minutes. Turn down the heat to medium or low so that it simmers. The liquid should be evaporated once the rice is cooked, and the rice should not be crunchy. Remove from heat and let the rice sit with the lid on for 10 minutes. Remove the lid, stir in the sriracha, and add lime to taste.

Egg Whites and Toast

This is a basic breakfast recipe with high protein and healthy carbohydrates. Substitutions can be made for mix-ins with the whites, such as salsa, avocado, or guacamole. Regular eggs can be used to add fats or for taste but will also add cholesterol.

Serves 2

Ingredients

- 2 cups egg whites
- 1 cup chopped multicolored peppers and onions
- 1 half teaspoon garlic powder
- 2 slices of multigrain toast
- 2 tablespoons jam or jelly
- 1 cup blueberries or another berry

1) Preheat a skillet to medium-high heat. Pour in peppers and onions and let them cook for 5-6 minutes before adding whites. After whites begin to solidify, mix in further with peppers and onions. Add in garlic powder. Continue to fluff the mixture until the eggs are solidified. Remove mixture from heat and separate into two servings.

2) Toast slices of multigrain bread to desired crispiness. Add a tablespoon of natural jelly to each.

3) Wash blueberries under cool water and drain. Divide into two and serve.

Other dish recommendations:

Grilled Mahi

Seared Steak

Grilled Shrimp

Roasted Turkey

Steamed Broccoli or Cauliflower

Riced Cauliflower -optional- mixed with peppers or spinach

Quinoa

Zucchini and Squash Medley

Side Salad -optional- chopped healthy protein mixed in

Chapter 8: Sample Routines

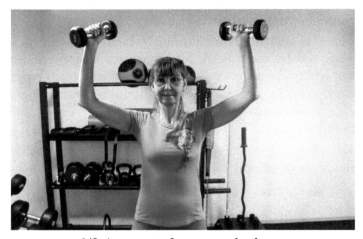

143. A woman performs an overhead press

The Big Lifts

Squats

Deadlifts

Overhead Press

Bench Press

Lat Pull Downs

These lifts should be first and foremost in your workouts, as they have the potential to use the most effort, muscles, and weight. These exercises should be the headliner of your workout routine for the day and the ones you want to try to hit every week.

While it is usually recommended to hit these exercises for around 3 sets of 10 reps if you must, you can lower these down to either 2 sets of 8 or 3 sets of 5. Getting these lifts in regularly will build overall strength and balance. While performing these movements, you will incorporate many other small or accessory muscles that will also benefit. Bodybuilding routines to enhance muscle growth usually include high rep numbers like 10 per set with 3-4 sets. For strength building, you can perform lower reps around 5-6 with around 5 sets.

Take the rest that you need to get the lift in. A workout can be long or short, but it should be effective. When you have the freedom and energy, take the time to have a complete workout with adequate rest between lifts to ensure you can perform the movements properly. If you don't have as much time or energy, cut the workout shorter by reducing the amount you are doing, not by reducing rest times. Rest times usually range from 30-60 seconds, depending on the weight of the exercise, how you are feeling, and whether the exercise is a big lift or not. A more extended rest period, such as 90 seconds-2 minutes, can be used when needed to ensure the lifts are performed.

When focusing on these large lifts, the other movements should come secondary and be performed afterward. The goal would be to get in every rep you aim to with good form for these big lifts. When you get to the other exercises and further into your workout, it is okay if you cannot perform the full number of sets or repetitions. Do what you can, and don't push it or risk injury. Recording your progress and what you've completed, such as sets, reps, time, and weight, can help you better address the next workout. You can always look back and spend more time on movements that didn't get addressed well earlier in the week.

Workouts should range from 15-45 minutes. It's important to strive for 30 minutes of good activity a day, but a hard workout can be 15 minutes with some chores or walking throughout the rest of the day. A long workout would be about 45 minutes and will likely require some resting later in the day. The duration of a workout should be based on how hard you are pushing and how much feels safe for you that day. Below are some sample routines that incorporate the entire body. On the off days you are not performing these, you will want to rest and stretch or perform yoga.

Full Body Routines

Warm-up: Wrists, Arms, Legs

Knee Pushup

Squat

Biceps Curl

Bent Lateral Raise

Arm Leg Raise

Warm-up: Legs, Shoulders, Back, Wrist

Deadlift

Front Raise

Overhead Triceps extension

Seated Row

Side bends

Warm-up: Back, Wrist, Arms, Chest

Bent Over Row

Bench Press

Calf Raises

Plank

Cable biceps curl

Warm-up: Shoulders, Arms, Legs, Wrists

Overhead Press

Dead bug

Straight Arm Pulldown

Lunge

Close-Grip Bench Press

Warm-up: Back, Shoulders, Chest, Wrist

Lat Pulldown

Wood Chop

Floor bridge

Chest Flys

Dips

Cardio

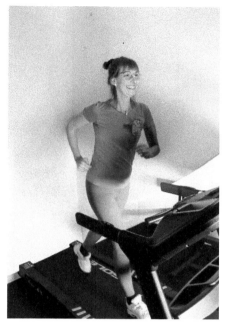

144. A senior on a run

This would be an example of a workout to perform focusing on cardio. During a week where you are only exercising a few days, this is what a cardio day would look like.

Warm-up: Legs, Back, Wrists

Walk, Bike or Dance

Plank

I, Y, T Raises

Warm-up: Legs, Back

Walk, Bike or Dance

Lat Pull Down

Dead Bug

Warm-up: Legs, Wrists, Chest, Back

Dance, Walk, Bike

Deadlift

Pushup

Arm Leg Raise

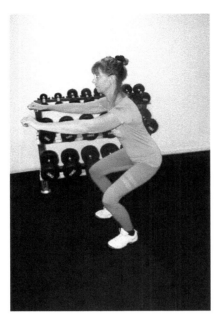

145. A senior doing a squat

Shortened or Strength-Focused Routines

These routines would be for working out fewer days during the week. These concentrate on big lifts that can be alternated week to week. Be sure to rest between lifts and use adequate weight as these workouts are shortened and more focused.

Warm-up: Wrists, Legs, Back

Squat/Bent Row

Plank

Dance

Warm-up: Wrists, Chest, Legs

Bench Press/Pushup

Floor Bridge

Walk

Warm-up: Legs, Back, Wrists

Deadlift/Pullup

Arm Leg Raise

Walk

Chapter 9: Balance, Energy, and Meditation

Seniors can have issues with balance that just naturally occur with being older. While this is common, it is still frightening, restrictive, and possibly dangerous. To combat this issue, seniors should stretch regularly. Staying loose and flexible can keep muscles from tightening up and causing falling issues. Keeping flexible can also help reduce the strain on joints that may interrupt their function.

As you age, the way you move changes based on your body changing over time. It's also harder to compensate when you trip or lean over when you're a senior because of these changes. It's best to be cognizant of these possibilities and address any issues you may have. Knowing what to expect and planning can help change whether you fall or not.

Medications, circulation, blood pressure, and less production of some nutrients can cause dizziness. These are all common issues for seniors and may happen occasionally or frequently. While some issues may be preventable by getting up slowly or taking medication and vitamins at the right time, others will occur when you least expect it. Since these things are possible, as a senior, you must do what you can to compensate physically. If you sense you are falling, not having the strength to catch yourself could lead to an unnecessary injury

Aside from regular stretching, you can perform some exercises to help build stability. These exercises can help move seamlessly in various directions and strengthen the core to help hold the body upright and brace for any unexpected movements. Lastly, exercises that target one side of the body or strengthen individual limbs can help provide extra balance and power to offset stability issues.

Balance Exercises

Sit-to-Stand

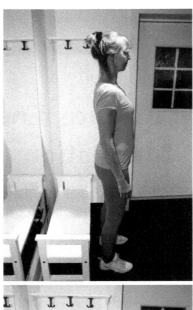

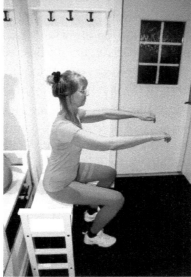

146. A woman performs sit-to-stand

1) Get a sturdy chair. Stand with your back facing it and feet hip-width apart. If you need to, you can hold onto something for support to get up and down but use this as a guide, not the primary source of power.

2) Sit back into the chair by pushing your hips back and slowly lowering them. Do this slowly to build strength. Pause once you are in the chair.

3) Stand back up by pushing through your heels without swinging or relying on your arms to push or push you up.

4) You should end in a standing position in front of the chair.

5) Perform 10 repetitions.

Shoulder Look Walking

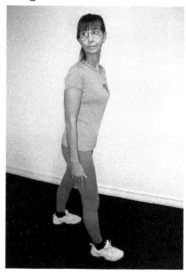

147. Woman performing shoulder look walking

1) Stand on one side of a room or straight hallway. Stand up with a straight back and shoulders back. If you need to, you can put your hand along the wall as you walk to keep you from falling.

2) Look over your shoulder and behind you moving only your head and neck.

3) Keep this position and take a few steps forward. Pause and look behind and over your other shoulder. Maintain this position and take a few steps forward.

4) Repeat this movement for 5 repetitions on each side.

Single Leg Stands

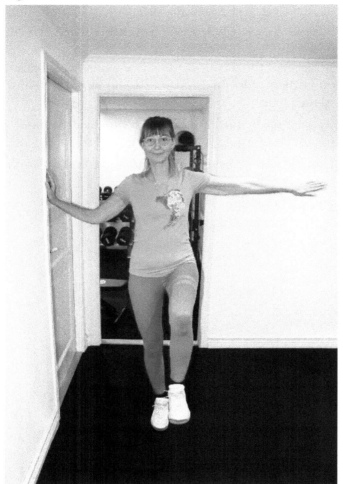

148. Seniors performing single leg stands

1) Stand with your feet hip-width apart. Keep your back straight and neck neutral. If you need to, use a wall or other object to keep your balance until you don't need it.

2) Lift your right foot a few inches off the floor. Do not let your body move, and don't lean to try to compensate. Hold this position and count to 10.

3) Return your foot to the floor.

4) Raise your left foot a few inches off the floor and repeat.

5) Perform this for 5 repetitions on each leg.

Standing March

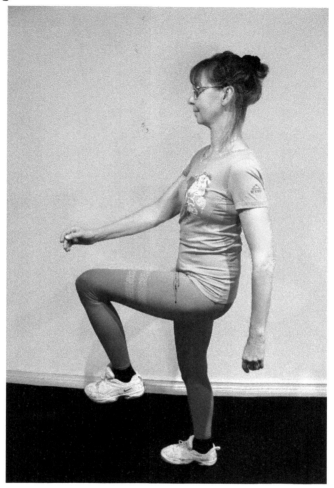

149. A woman performs the standing march

1) Stand with your feet hip-width apart. Keep your back straight and neck neutral.

2) Lift one knee until your thigh is parallel to the ground. Pause briefly at the top. Do not lean or bend to compensate. You can hold a chair, counter, or wall to keep your balance until you no longer need to.

3) Slowly return your leg back down to the ground.

4) Switch legs and repeat.

5) Perform 10 marches on each side while alternating legs.

Heel Toe Walk

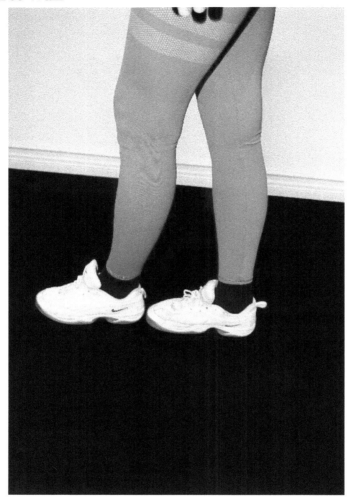

150. An exerciser walking heel to toe

1) Stand with back straight and shoulders back.

2) Step with your left foot slightly in front of you. Place the right foot directly behind it so the toes touch your left heel. Your feet should always be toe-to-heel when placed on the floor during this exercise.

3) Move your right foot in front of your left without moving the left.

4) Repeat with the left foot.

5) Complete this for 10 steps with each foot.

Balance Reach

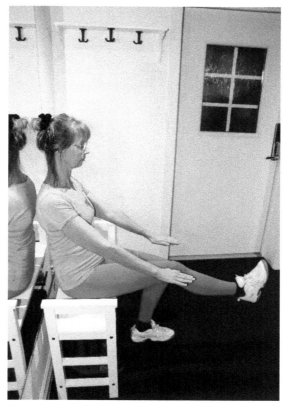

151. A senior performs a seated single-leg balance and reach

1) Stand facing the back of a chair. Hold onto the chair with your left hand.

2) Lift your right leg and extend your right arm straight out in front of you at shoulder height. Pause.

3) While holding this position move your extended arm to your right until it is straight out to your side. Pause

4) Bring your extended arm straight behind you, so it points opposite your left. This position should be opposite of the direction your extended arm began in. Pause.

5) Return your extended arm back to the side position. Pause

6) Return your extended arm straight out in front of you. Pause.

7) Switch arms and legs and repeat.

8) Perform this entire process two times on each side.

Side and Rear Leg Raise

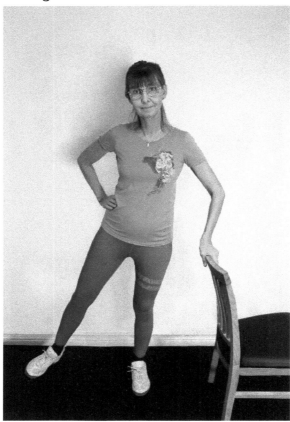

152. A woman performs side leg raises

1) Stand behind the back of a sturdy chair with your feet slightly apart. Hold onto the chair with one or both hands for support. Keep your back straight and neck neutral.

2) Slowly lift your left leg straight out to the side left side. Your toes will remain facing forward. Only your leg should move. Raise it until you feel comfortable. Pause.

3) Lower the leg back down.

4) Raise the leg again straight back behind you, keeping it as straight as possible. Pause.

5) Return to start.

6) Switch legs and repeat.

7) Perform this exercise 12 times per leg.

Breathing

Breathing, like the exercises used in yoga, is helpful for many other situations. Breathing can be used to reduce anxiety, improve sleep, or even help power you through moving a heavy object. Regularly practicing breathing exercises will eventually improve your breathing in usable real-life situations. Below are breathing practices you can use to help you in various situations to maintain mental balance, boost energy, and find peace.

Breathing Exercises

Warm-up Breathing

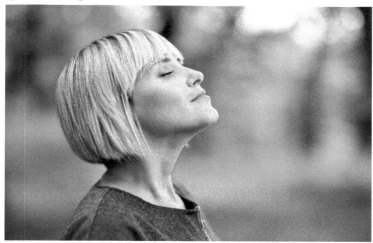

153. A woman focused on breathing

Use this technique to warm up before other breathing exercises, a stretching session, or the beginning of the workout. This is a quick exercise to get you focused on the task at hand.

1) Sit or stand with your back straight, chest up, shoulders back, and neck neutral.

2) Inhale slowly through your nose for at least a count of 4 as you focus on only your breath coming in and your lungs and chest rising.

3) Breathe out through your mouth again slowly for at least 8 seconds. Focus on pushing the air out and your lungs emptying. Your chest should fall as you breathe out.

4) Repeat this for 1 minute.

Pursed Lip Breathing

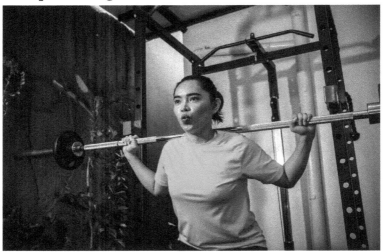

154. A woman uses pursed lip breathing while lifting

This method can help those who smoke or are inactive improve their lung capacity. This technique improves the lungs' ability to take quality breaths.

1) Sit or stand with your back straight, chest up, shoulders back, and neck neutral.

2) Breathe in deeply through your nose and try to fill your lungs. Focus on getting the air into your body and feeling it fill your lungs.

3) Pause and hold your breath for at least a full second

4) Purse your lips (make them firm in the shape they would be in while using a small straw)

5) Breathe out slowly from your pursed lips for at least 6 seconds. Try to get all the air out without forcing it. Keep your mouth pursed and concentrate on your lungs, expelling the air.

6) This exercise can be repeated for up to ten minutes.

Work Breathing

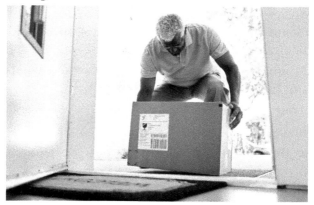

155. A senior picking up a box

This method is used when lifting a heavy object or during any type of physical exertion.

1) Stand before the object you are about to lift with a straight back and neutral neck.

2) Inhale deeply through your nose.

3) As you lift the object or exert force, breathe out through your mouth with pursed lips (when the lips are held firmly in a position like you are using a small straw).

4) Breathe normally once the effort has been exerted.

Deep Breaths

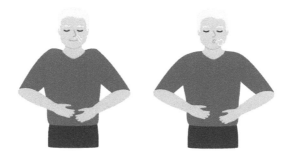

156. A man practices deep breathing

This is a calming technique using breathing. You can use this to help relieve anxiety.

1) Sit or stand with your back straight, chest up, shoulders back, and neck neutral.

2) Breathe in through your nose for at least 6 seconds. Pull the air into your lungs and down deep to your belly.

3) Hold your breath for at least 2 seconds.

4) Breathe out for at least an 8 count.

5) Repeat this method at least 10 times. Rest for 1 minute with regular breathing between exercises.

Calm Breathing

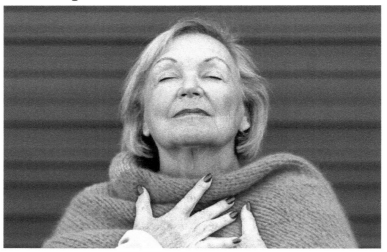

157. A woman uses calm breathing

This exercise should be used to set the mind and body at ease. Use this to slow your breathing and help you focus.

1) Sit or stand with your back straight, chest up, shoulders back, and neck neutral.

2) Inhale slowly for a count of 2, to begin with. Pause and hold your breath.

3) Exhale slowly for a count of 2.

4) You can increase this exercise's difficulty by counting to higher numbers on both the inhale and exhale.

Deep Quick Breathing

This method will quickly lower your heart rate and blood pressure. It can be used to calm you down when you are stressed, panicked, or overexerted from physical activity.

1) Sit or stand with your back straight, chest up, shoulders back, and neck neutral.

2) Inhale deeply through your nose and feel your lungs filling with air. Feel the air flow down through your lungs into your belly.

3) Breathe out normally for a count of 8 through your mouth.

4) Repeat this until you feel calm or for up to five minutes.

Nose Breathing

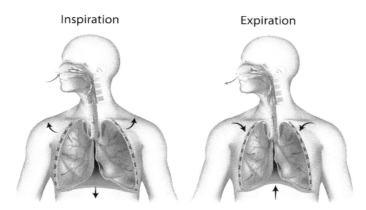

Inspiration   Expiration

158. A model of the body using nose breathing

You can use this method to help you catch your breath. This technique is for those trying to use each breath better, utilizing their nose and lungs.

Sit or stand with your back straight, chest up, shoulders back, and neck neutral.

1) Breathe in through your nose for about a 4 count

2) Breathe out through your nose until all the air is expelled from your body.

3) Slow down your breathing and continue to breathe in and out through your nose in this fashion. Each time you should be slightly increasing your breaths in and out.

4) Focus on getting air in through your nose and using it. Then focus on letting it all back out. Do not push, but rather try to remain calm during this technique.

Meditation

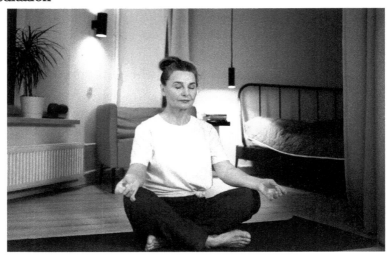
159. A senior practicing meditation

Meditation is the practice of preparing your body and mind to deal with specific situations, thoughts, and feelings. It's a training method just like exercise that works out your mind and spirit. It is used to help you stay balanced and live life as positively as possible. Meditation improves concentration, reduces stress, builds beneficial habits, and boosts discipline.

Meditation can help seniors solve problems, improve sleep, and even manage pain. Instead of sulking, letting dark days linger, or giving in to urges like snacking, seniors can use meditation as a tool to empower themselves. Meditation simply requires habitual practice so that when a challenging situation arises, you can tap into your meditation mindset easily

Meditation can be broken down into two main divisions. The techniques may seem overly simple, but the more you give yourself over to them and believe in their effectiveness, the better they will work.

Open meditation requires you to open up your awareness. It asks you to be in the moment and focus on all aspects of your environment. During this process, you should acknowledge and analyze your thoughts, thought process, how you feel about yourself, how your *self* exists in the current situation, and all your current impulses and feelings at the moment.

Focused meditation asks you to focus on a single aspect of the moment. This technique requires pushing everything else to the side; therefore, you are purely concentrating on a single thing. During this process, you can focus on a sound, thought, object, breathing, mantra, or saying.

To practice these, you will need to find somewhere quiet to truly focus on them. When you use these meditations later, they may not always be in a quiet place -- which is why practice is required to instill them firmly. It is recommended to start first thing in the morning so that your day begins with an insightful and uplifting practice.

Relaxing Activities

Deep Breathing – Practice focusing on each breath going in and out. Use the breathing techniques listed in the section above.

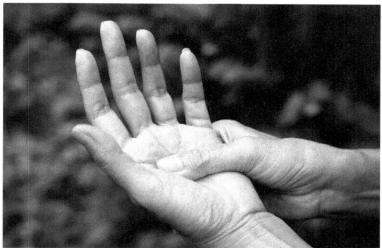

160. A self-hand massage

Massage – You can massage your own legs, feet, hips, neck, shoulders, arms, and hands or have someone else do it for you. Apply pressure so that it feels comforting and take the time to really work on the area you are massaging.

Yoga – Yoga can boost energy or relax the body depending on how you approach it and what moves you perform.

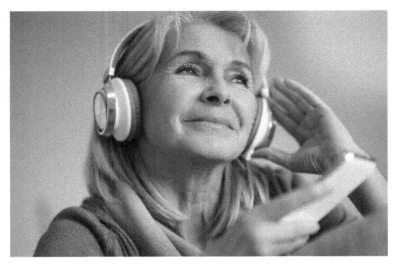

161. A senior listening to music

Listening or making Music – Music can calm you down, help you focus, or transport you to another time and place.

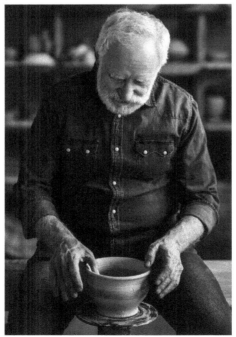

162. A senior doing pottery

Looking at (or creating) Art – Art can help you focus on a particular place or time and take you away from where you currently are.

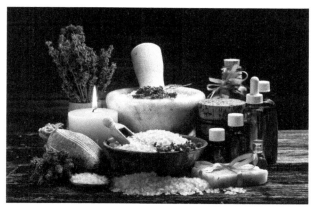
163. A collection of aromatherapy implements

Pleasant Aromas – Candles or lotions can provide smells that take you away or entirely change your emotional state.

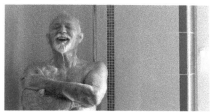
164. A senior enjoying a shower

Taking a Bath or Shower – Take a leisurely bath or shower and try to find joy in getting yourself clean. The warm water and steam it creates can relax your muscles and clear your mind.

Visualizing – See a place by closing your eyes and trying to transport yourself fully there. Try to engage all your senses in this transportation.

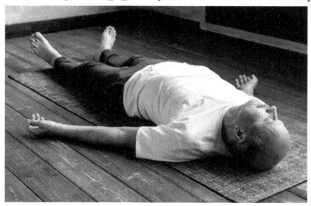
165. A senior lying down and relaxing muscles

Relax your muscles – Slowly, one by one, focus on relaxing your muscles. An excellent position to practice this is lying flat on your back with your spine fully extended and your body completely flat.

Mantras – Repeat a phrase or word over and over while calming your mind by focusing on what you are trying to accomplish. You can also slow your breathing as you speak to calm your heart rate further.

Chapter 10: Sharpening the Sword

You now have a complete text packed with exercises, diet tips, strategies for managing mental health, and the benefits of using these. This book provides you with the information you need, with details on how to use it to help yourself. Your curiosity should be adequately piqued by all the potential goodness you can experience by following the recommendations in this book. Understandably, motivation may still be an issue.

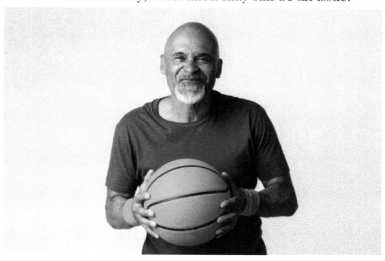

166. A senior holding a basketball

Motivation is not something that comes easy for everyone, and there are many ways to talk yourself out of doing something. This text has some motivation based on personal experiences with seniors. The truth, though, is that it will be up to you to finally act once you've read through or repeatedly skimmed through this book. It's up to you to try it, even if it is only a little try. All that can be promised is that this book intends to help you. So, following these diet tips, exercising, or even just experimenting with yoga should do just that. Hopefully, after your first attempts, you will experience benefits that trigger you to proceed with adopting an exercise lifestyle.

To help improve these chances and make exercising more interesting, you can do a few things. Make exercise a part of your life. Schedule time for exercise and devote a little of yourself to it daily. It shouldn't be a burden but something that you look forward to either because of how you feel afterward or because it's an escape from your regular routine.

Let others know about your exercise journey as well. Tell your friends and family about your goals or what you did for your workout yesterday. Yes, they want to know because if it's something that's helping you, it will also make them happy.

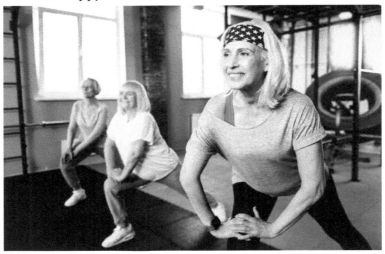
167. Seniors exercising together

Once you get going, you can invite your friends or family to participate. Meeting up with a buddy for your workouts is not only fun, but it also helps hold you accountable. Use the support system you have around you, or if you don't have one create it through exercise. You can join a gym, a run club, or a morning walk group. These social groups will give you someone to swap stories with or compete with when it comes to exercise. This interaction can become a source of motivation or something you look forward to daily, weekly, or monthly.

Having an exercise buddy or working out at the gym is also a way to look out for your safety. Everybody makes mistakes, and it's nice to have someone there to help you out when you do. Seniors are more susceptible to injury from reduced muscle mass, stiff joints, and decreases in bone density. This doesn't mean you should hide in a bubble; you must take action to combat these things. At the same time, be aware of them and make intelligent choices like exercising with a buddy.

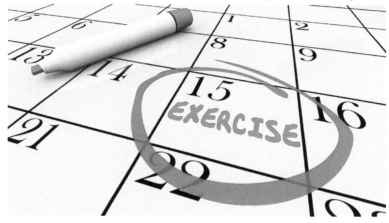

168. An exercise calendar

Keep track of your exercise. Putting all your work on paper or a computer will make it even more worthwhile. You'll be able to see all that you've done and even share it with others. Having a record of your exercise is almost like having a report of all your visits with a doctor. They are valuable and informative to you and anyone else who may see them, like a trainer or healthcare provider.

Keeping track of your exercise can also keep you going. Marking on the calendar, for example, what type of workout you do each day can build a habit. Then when you look back at all the marked days, you realize you've been working hard for months! Staying consistent is essential; the more you exercise, the more you will benefit. Remember, even if you only do a little each day, staying active will impact you.

Once you reach a plateau and exercise becomes boring or too easy, it's time to change things. There are plenty of ways to increase the difficulty of exercises. Each change you make will add a new and different aspect to the results of your efforts. Add more weight, try a single limb instead of double, or choose a different exercise entirely as a substitute. Make sure you keep exercise fun and interesting because it can be, and for a senior enjoying your life, it should be.

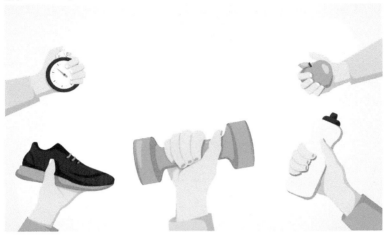

169. Hands holding exercise essentials

Take your curiosity and desire to reduce your joint pain, lose weight or sleep better and use this book to do it. Do it for yourself and do it for your loved ones. You never know what effect exercising may have on your life. It may decrease your trips to the doctor, reduce your medications, or lift a cloud that's been looming over your head.

Fighting for yourself by exercising and eating better may also rub off on others. If there's someone you want to help or change, lead by example and show them what being a healthy senior can look like!

Part 2: Resistance Band Workout for Seniors

The Only Workout Program with Resistance Bands You'll Ever Need

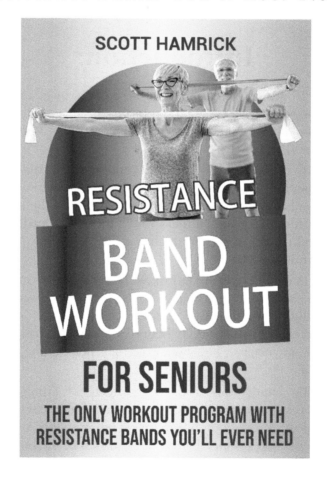

Introduction:

One in every 10 adults over the age of 60 rapidly loses muscle strength with each passing year. The first symptoms of losing strength are the constant feeling of tiredness, aching body pain, and becoming slower when participating in physical activity.

But the thing is that losing strength is completely normal. The average middle-aged person loses up to 3-8% of muscle mass every decade. Muscle loss is also believed to have a big impact on the stability of the joints. Lack of muscle causes stiffness which inevitably leads to joint pain. If left untreated, it can affect the quality of life. Extreme cases can even lead to losing independence.

Of course, being able to run and move heavy things around seems like a superhuman ability after reaching your 60s. But what if you were able to gain that so-called "superhuman" ability back? Well, the good news is... you absolutely can. And the even better news is that you can do it for free... anytime, anywhere. The big secret lies behind the power of the resistance band.

These elastic bands have the same effects as lifting free weights. Combining a resistance band with a couple of exercises rebuilds the muscle mass lost throughout the years. The way this works is pretty simple. When using resistance bands, the muscles in the body go through hypertrophy. This is when the fiber of the muscles gets broken down from the tension applied from the resistance bands.

Technically speaking, the muscles get damaged and ripped. Although this might sound like a bad thing, it's the only way to grow back new muscle and increase strength. Following a 20-minute resistance band workout with good rest and a balanced diet will eventually make these damaged muscles "heal."

The healing process includes new muscle mass developing in these "ripped" areas. The reason why it's so simple to build new muscle is that it takes even the lightest of exercise for hypertrophy to take place.

As surprising as it might seem, rebuilding strength as a senior is not the hard part. The hard part is consistency. Being determined to grab that resistance band is hard. Not because the exercises are too exhausting, or because they are too confusing... NO. Actually, 97% of people admit to feeling their best after a resistance band workout.

The real scientific reason why being consistent is hard is due to the mind precepting this new activity as something strange and unusual. It's not yet part of the daily routine, so both the mind and body try to avoid it at all costs. Now, what happens is that the mind makes 1000 excuses to skip that 20-minute exercise, even though it is conscious of all the long-term benefits. But the thing is, that once you defeat the mind's excuses telling you to skip that workout, you are setting yourself up for effortless success!

The following chapters of this book will not only touch on every aspect of how to build strength and ease muscle pain, but it will also give you a higher ability to persuade your mind on being consistent.

Reminder: The purpose of this book is only to inform and educate readers. It is NOT intended to act as a substitute for curing illnesses or medical diagnoses. DO NOT use this book to get self-diagnosed or self-treated. Always contact your doctor before taking medication, changing your eating habits, or start including a workout in your daily routine.

Chapter 1: The Power of the Resistance Band:

In 1895 a philanthropist named Gustav Gossweiler patented his idea of weird gym equipment for that era. The invention was a stretchy elastic band that would increase muscle resistance during a workout session.

More than a century later, Gossweiler's invention would be used for numerous purposes. Whether it is to ease arthritic pain, gain mobility, reduce the risk of losing balance, or gain back muscle mass. Physical therapists and professional trainers have been recommending resistance bands to their clients for decades. This is because resistance bands have shown to be 2x times more effective than lifting free weights.

For example, when using a 2-pound dumbbell to do a bicep curl, the muscle uses the same amount of resistance from the moment you raise the dumbbell until the curl is finalized. Another thing about free weights is that it doesn't provide continuous muscle tension. As you lower the dumbbell after finishing a biceps curl, it stops further stimulating the muscle. This occurs because the dumbbell is no longer being pulled down by gravity while you drop it to starting position.

On the other hand, holding on to a resistance band with one hand and pulling it with the other will have a completely different impact on the muscle. The more the band is pulled, the more resistance it causes. This happens because, unlike free weights, resistance bands do not solely rely on gravity. In addition, bands put the muscle under constant tension when being used.

With free weights, you can only exercise effectively on a vertical plane. So, say if you were to hold a dumbbell and move it left and right, it would have no effect on the muscle. Relying on gravity is the biggest weak point of free weights as it limits the movement of the body.

Resistance bands give users the freedom of moving their entire body while exercising. A workout using these bands can go as far as allowing your body to twist, sidekick, swing, and bend. Taking different positions while adding resistance to the muscles boosts flexibility and balance while reducing body stiffness and joint pain.

If you're not sure where to start or what type of program would be right for you, this book will help you make a decision. We'll look at some of the benefits of exercising as a senior, as well as some tips on how to stay motivated throughout your fitness journey.

Step 1. Starting your journey

Start slowly and gradually increase your exercise intensity. The more you can do, the better. Start with at least 20 minutes of aerobic or full body workout on 4 to 5 days of the week. This can be done in the comfort of your own home with a resistance band workout routine. If you have not been exercising regularly, start with shorter periods and gradually increase the duration over several weeks until you can exercise at least 30 minutes on most days of the week (or whatever target you set).

Strength training exercises should be done 2 to 3 times a week and should include exercises that work all major muscle groups in your body. Your initial goal should be 10 reps per set. As you get stronger, increase the number of reps until you reach about 15 per set for most exercises (but lower this number if needed).

Step 2 Making the exercise routine, a routine!

In this stage, your goal is to continue with your exercise program at an intensity that is appropriate for your current fitness level. You will still see physical changes because of maintaining a regular exercise routine. The difference is that now you can increase the frequency of your workouts. It is important to remember that even though this stage does not

require as much attention as beginning to workout, it still requires effort on your part.

Step 3 Maintaining

The maintenance stage is an important one because it helps you to maintain the benefits of your exercise program. You have been exercising for 6 months or longer and are continuing to do so as part of your lifestyle.

During this time, you may begin to notice that some of your initial improvements have started to show significantly. These are all natural changes that happen to everyone who exercises regularly. When you're in the maintenance stage, it's important to keep up with your regular exercise schedule as best as possible — so that the problems you once had don't get worse again!

Obstacles

While thinking about your motivations, you will want to consider possible obstacles and plan ways to overcome them. The most common barriers for older adults seem to be:

Lack of time: It's hard to find time for exercise when there is so much else going on in your life. One way around this problem is to schedule regular exercise sessions in your weekly routine. For example, if you know that every Tuesday at 6 pm you're busy with other activities, don't schedule a workout session then! Try scheduling it at 5 pm or 7 pm instead. If necessary, break up your workout into several short sessions throughout the day instead of one long session at the end of the day. Most people find it better to complete a workout first thing in the morning as it not only boosts their energy for the rest of the day, but they also feel less tired than when doing them during the afternoon or evening.

Another reason is that you might think it's too hard or tiring. Well, it's supposed to be! If it wasn't challenging, we wouldn't get any benefit from it. But if you have a goal in mind–such as losing weight–then the exercise will help achieve that goal. The more often you exercise, the easier it gets. You'll notice that it becomes part of your lifestyle and routine after a while. Your body will also adapt so that some activities seem easier than when you first started doing them.

Fear of injury: Many people avoid exercising because they think they might injure themselves if they try something new or do it incorrectly. If you follow proper guidelines when exercising and make sure that everything feels comfortable before proceeding to more difficult movements, your risk of injury should be minimal.

Fear of embarrassment. Maybe you're afraid of being laughed at or ridiculed by others because they might see how out-of-shape (or old) you are compared with other people in their age group of your social circle.

Or perhaps they'll just think that everyone else has better bodies than you do — which isn't true anyway! It helps to remember that everyone starts somewhere and has different levels of fitness; there's no need to compare yourself with anyone else!.

Overcoming Obstacles

If you feel stressed out and tired all the time, try this simple technique: Close your eyes and visualize yourself exercising. Imagine yourself running on a beach or doing yoga at the mountains, climbing stairs in a skyscraper, or resistance band training at a comfortable spot in your home. This visualization technique is often used by athletes to prepare for an important competition or event—it helps them mentally prepare for what they have to do physically. You can use it too!

In 1998, the American Journal of Sports Medicine conducted a study about the effectiveness of elastic bands in tennis players. The study showed that out of all the professional tennis players, the ones that consistently used resistance bands in their workout routine had a better ball throwing speed and enhanced shoulder strength compared to players that didn't include bands in their training.

Its high effectiveness and easy-to-use nature make the resistance band the ideal equipment for beginners, people who work out at home, and seniors. They are cost-effective and suitable to fit any lifestyle (even for the most frequent of travelers). Resistance bands come in three shapes:

1. Loop Bands

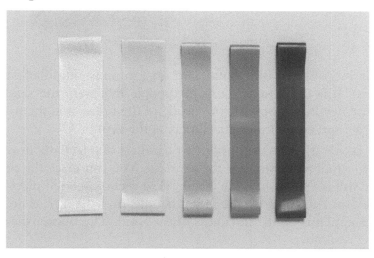

Loop bands have a flat and rubber band-like appearance. They are used mainly for strengthening the lower leg muscles and the upper arms and shoulders.

There are 3 ways to wear the loop band. The most common way is by putting both of your legs inside the band and raising them two inches above your knees. You can also keep the band right above ankle length.

Using a loop band for the lower body works mainly with your glutes. Other secondary muscles that get put to work are the quadriceps, calves, hamstrings, and trunk.

For upper body use, put the loop band around both your arms at wrist length. The colors of the tubes determine the level of resistance the band provides. Usually, the lighter the color of the band the lighter the resistance.

2. Tube bands

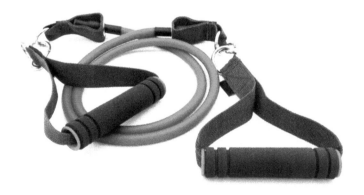

Unlike loop bands, tube bands are set to mimic dumbbells and gym equipment. It is the best solution for people that want the same results without the need of stepping foot outside of the house and the troubles of lifting heavy and complicated machinery at the gym.

Tube bands usually come with two handles; one to hang in place and the other to pull and complete the exercise. You can place the tube band wherever you see fit around the house. Best recommended place that will keep the band intact is at the door handle or a hanger. The level of resistance depends on the thickness of the band. The thicker the tube the higher the resistance.

3. Thera bands

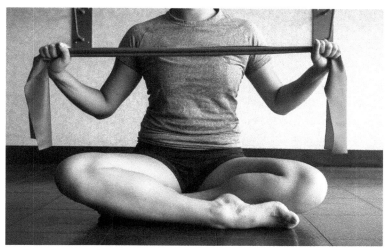

These bands are also known as light therapy bands as they are great if you are trying to gain mobility from an injury or due to age complications. They are highly recommended if you are suffering from body stiffness and joint pain. These bands are light, which makes them perfect for people that want a low-impact workout that delivers results without much resistance.

Thera bands usually range from 6 to 8 feet long. Its length is great for stretching and improving flexibility. The bands work on most muscles in the body by stretching and lightly toning them.

If you are a beginner at using bands, it is recommended to start with a thera band that has a light to medium resistance difficulty. Beginners should be completing an average of 2 hours of light physical activity every week. Two out of seven days should include resistance band workouts with thera bands.

When training with the band as a beginner, the exercise session should last 10-20 minutes. It is important to start slow and awaken the muscles gradually without causing too much trauma. A huge problem with most beginners getting into resistance band exercises is that they get the "rush of the start" where they feel highly motivated and try to double or even triple the amount of activity from the very first few sessions. Some even go as far as using high-difficulty resistance bands right from the start because they believe that will help them reach their goal faster.

But, the truth is far from this belief. Not taking things slowly will just lead to massive muscle aches for the next few days. In most cases when this happens, the body is too sore and tired to do the next day's workout. This increases the chances of being inconsistent and eventually skipping physical activity altogether.

Another reason why starting heavy is not recommended is because it can be fatal. Using a short loop band or a tube band from the very beginning can oftentimes lead to injury. This is because these bands are shorter and put more resistance to the muscle. If the muscles aren't used to it, they can get easily exhausted and let go of the band, causing them to hit the body and injure it. This is comparable to two people pulling a rubber band from opposite ends. When one of them lets go of holding it, the rubber band hits the other person, leaving them in massive pain.

When starting with resistance bands, always be sure to listen to your body. Immediately stop working out if you start feeling dizzy and lightheaded. That stands true when you also feel uneasy, sick, or uncomfortable during the workout. Another time when you should stop exercising is when you feel pain. Although it is normal to feel a slight burn in the muscle area you are stimulating, feeling any other type of pain is not normal.

If any of these three cases happen during a resistance band workout, make sure to talk to a healthcare provider to see if you are physically able to continue using bands in your workout routine.

As your body strengthens in time, you can start to add the difficulty level of the thera band and add a short loop band with the lightest resistance level. Depending on the strength gained after the first few months, you can also try different resistance band shapes and difficulty levels to find which one is the best fit for you. There are three main reasons why you should use resistance bands over the age of 60:

Increased mobility

The biggest problem older adults face is the fact that they start getting stiffer. Getting out of bed in the morning or trying to move after sitting for a long time can feel like a challenge.

These feelings of restriction eventually get eased as the muscles warm up as soon as they start moving. But in most cases, even after the body warms up, the feeling of flexibility is not as close as what it used to be back in the old days. The reason mobility decreases as the body ages are linked to many factors.

The most common reason is age-associated conditions. Some of them include osteoporosis, which is a condition where the bones of the body get significantly reduced in mass and eventually become brittle, osteoarthritis, which happens when the cartilage in the joints gets damaged and osteomalacia which is a condition where the bones get brittle due to the lack of vitamin D in the body.

Although these are three of the most common conditions that impact mobility in adults over 60, the most popular one people face as they age is sarcopenia. The condition causes the bones and muscles of the body to weaken without an external cause. Some symptoms of sarcopenia are loss of mobility, muscle weakness, inflammation of joints, and rheumatoid arthritis.

Unfortunately, studies show that age-related conditions are not the only cause of loss of mobility. Blood also plays a big part. As the body ages, the arteries of the body become stiffer. This stiffness leads to more blood going to the feet. The lack of blood flow in other areas of the body inevitably leads the muscles to weaken.

Another contributing factor to the loss of mobility is the loss of flexibility of ligaments. These are tendons that are naturally relaxed during early adulthood. The main cause of ligaments losing flexibility is the lack of movement of the body over the years.

The good thing is that age-related conditions and complications that cause body stiffness can easily be reduced or even prevented with the use of resistance bands. To maintain or even gain the lost mass over the years, muscles need to be frequently stimulated and put to use. The same is true for the bones. In order to maintain or gain bone density, the bone needs constant stimulation.

When using resistance bands, not only do the muscles and bones get stimulated, but the cartilage of the joints gets put to work more often. When active, the cartilage brings in synovial fluid which makes the movement of the joints easier. Using resistance bands also increases the blood flow throughout the body as it stretches and moves the arteries.

Back in the day, trainers used to motivate their clients to work out by telling them: "Either move it or lose it." That saying also stands true for adults over 60, because you can either decide to stay slightly active and keep your body from disuse or continue losing mobility on higher levels.

Prevent Injury

Falls are the major cause of injury and even death for seniors. In fact, falling and getting injured after is highly common. Based on the Center for Disease Control and Prevention, one in every four senior Americans falls and gets injured every year. This leads to an average of 36 million falls per year.

Unfortunately, out of these 36 million falls, 8 million of them result in serious injuries that require hospitalization. The most frequent injuries include the breaking of the hip, trauma to the head, and a breaking of the arms and legs. Falling and injuries leave tens of thousands of seniors to lose their mobility permanently.

Out of all the age groups, people that are 65 years or older are the most prone to get injured during an accident. Age-related conditions increase the chances of getting injured. Since the bones of the body become more brittle with age, there is a higher chance they can break during a fall. The lack of muscle in the body also increases the chances of accidents occurring. Feeling weak and restricted in body movement will make it more challenging to "think fast" before falling.

When falling, adults in their 20s and 30s have a much better grip to hold on to something to prevent a fall. This is all linked to the fact that they have more muscle mass and joint flexibility. This comparison was made having taken in mind that no matter what, the difference in health between both group ages is significantly different.

But the point stays at the ability to prevent injury. Stimulating and gaining lost muscle mass and bone mass by working out with resistance bands will give your body a better grip to hold on to a nearby object and prevent the fall.

Promote Weight Loss

A lot of people struggle to maintain or lose weight as they get older. And the thing is that many of these people have the same eating habits as they did decades ago, yet they still gain a few extra pounds.

Well, as a person grows older, they burn fewer calories when they are in a sedentary state. This means that doing things like blinking, yawning, and breathing require less energy to continue functioning normally.

Another reason that causes weight gain is that the body's metabolism gets slower. A slower metabolism no longer requires a lot of food. Something that makes gaining weight an even faster process after your 60s is the fact that working out and keeping the body active reduces.

But if this wasn't enough, older adults experience a shift in body composition with each passing year. This shift comes with muscle loss due to an inconsistent or nonexistent workout routine over the years. While the muscle mass reduces, fat mass replaces it. When this occurs, not only do you gain more body fat, but since fat is more metabolically active than muscles are, the body is no longer in need of "that much" food to maintain its weight.

What also causes weight gain with age is the hormonal changes in both men and women. Men lose testosterone levels which causes them to lose drastic muscle mass and therefore store more fat as a replacement. On the other hand, women go through menopause and have changes in many of their hormone levels, which eventually causes weight gain.

Before getting on to the workout, talk to a nutrition specialist or to your local healthcare provider about the amount of caloric intake your body needs to stop gaining weight. The best way to shed these few extra pounds and keep them off is by combining resistance band exercises with cardio exercises. A great routine would be by working out 5 times a week, with 3 times being a 15-20 minute light cardio workout and 2 times being a 20-minute resistance band workout.

Chapter 2: Rehab: Upper Body Pain

Rehab comes in many forms and techniques, but it all leads to the same purpose, which is to maintain or regain day-to-day life abilities. Rehab or better known as rehabilitation improves physical, mental, or even the ability to learn and think more efficiently.

People that seek rehab often have lost one of these abilities due to an injury, disease, or addiction. The reason why it's so popular in today's society is due to it being highly effective for thousands of years.

The earliest proof of rehab treatments was found in ancient China, known as the Cong Fu physical therapy movement. Dating thousands of years back, the Chinese would use rehabilitation to relieve pain caused by injury and disease. Evidence also suggests that the methods would be used by seniors experiencing rapid loss of mobility.

Greeks and Romans also started popularizing rehab around 500 BC - 200 AD. Greek physician Herodicus and Roman physician Galen massively contributed to modernizing and shaping rehab as it is known today. Both physicians believed in the benefits that gymnastic exercises bring to people suffering from physical complications.

These methods were further improved during the 1500s, by philologist-physician Mercurialis. Mercurialis published one of the first medical books ever to be written for rehab called "The Art of Gymnastics" in 1569. He heavily believed that aside from improving physical abilities, people could also prevent them by performing gymnastic exercises consistently.

The 18th century was followed by a boom in science and technology. During this time, Niels Stenson and Joseph Clement Tissot both researched the biometrics of human mobility and came up with a rather surprising discovery for the time. The scientists saw how fast people would heal from a physical injury in two very different conditions.

In one condition, injured patients had to stay on bed rest until recovery, while in the other condition, patients were encouraged to move their bodies through a certain set of physical activities.

The discovery revealed that the patients that performed physical activity after the injury, healed much faster than the ones placed on bed rest. There was also a big difference in mobility between patients who were bed rested and the ones that underwent rehab.

There were clear signs that the injured patients that were on bed rest had lost more mobility while the ones in physical rehab were performing much better, sometimes resulting in better shape than they were before they were injured. This study led Joseph Clement Tissot to publish the book Medical and Surgical Gymnastics in 1780 which would help further popularize rehab even in the western culture.

Rehab is a lengthy process and similar to weight loss, seeing results takes time and dedication. There are three stages the body goes through by using resistance bands as a physical rehab treatment.

The recovery phase.

Unlike the other two stages, recovery is the longest to overcome. This is because it's where the body starts "understanding" that changes are being made to it. Yet again, this is easily comparable to how the body reacts when on a diet. It doesn't start losing body fat right away, but it first starts understanding that changes are being made and starts burning glycogen stored in the liver and muscle before moving forward to excess water weight.

The recovery stage is quite a delicate phase as the body needs to start slowly adapting to the new stretches and exercises. If overdone, muscles or tendons can experience a strain. Strains happen when the muscles and tendons tear or get pulled too much from sudden unexpected activity. Not warming up the body before each physical activity session can also increase the chances of experiencing muscle strains.

Putting too much effort and intensity into the band exercises during the recovery phase might only cause trauma to the body and damage it even more. That is why starting slow is better. During this phase, the body is healing, so it needs a lot of rest. To say the least, the main focus of rehab is not to exercise to tire the body but to stretch it enough for the body to "wake up" and then give it the desired amount of rest to heal.

Resting doesn't always mean lying in bed or on the couch. It also includes applying heat or cold packs to areas that cause pain, reducing stress, keeping peace of mind, avoiding arguments or heated situations, and eating easier-to-digest food.

The repairing phase

After the body has fully adapted to the stretches and physical exercises using the bands, it starts becoming ready to repair itself. This stage is where the body starts gaining some flexibility and becomes less stiff. What happens is that your body tries to recover as much as it can back to how it was before.

The repairing stage is also delicate, which means that the band stretches and exercises should not be overdone. It is advised to stay away from tiring strength training during this time as the body is still in the healing phase. On the other hand, resting as much as before can slowly start being reduced.

Regaining back strength

When the body has restored the painful and stiff areas as much as it could, it is time to include strength exercises in the picture. Increased disuse of the body over the years and the resting phase of rehab both have contributed to the weakening of the muscles.

Now that the body has gotten used to the light resistance band workout you can finally start using heavier bands such as the loop and the tube bands, which add more resistance to the muscles. Also adding new strength exercises to your workout routine will tremendously help in completing this stage successfully.

Rehabilitation is highly important for ages 60 and above as they not only recover physical abilities lost over the years but also prevent further loss of these abilities. Seniors that are most in need of physical rehabilitation are ones suffering from side effects from medical treatments, underwent surgery, or suffer from age progressing conditions and chronic pain.

One of the most frequent problems older adults suffer from is chronic body pain. Body pain is common in almost every individual and varies from person to person. Chronic pain is when an individual suffers from a certain type of body pain for longer than 3 months.

If left untreated, chronic pain can reduce the quality of life and also lead to a loss of mobility in some cases. Three of the most common upper body pain people suffer from are neck, shoulder, and back pain. Keep in mind that when suffering from any type of upper and lower body pain, the body is considered injured.

Injury is only healed through rehabilitation and NOT by strength exercises. Trying to reduce the pain by immediately starting a workout routine might only increase the pain you might be experiencing. Instead, the best thing to do when experiencing pain, stiffness, or weakness in the body is to start slowly with corrective body stretches.

One out of every three seniors has suffered from neck pain at least once. Statistically, women are more prone to develop neck pain than men. This chronic pain only worsens with age. Most people describe neck pain as a constant and irritating feeling around the upper part of the neck or a feeling of tension in the neck muscles.

The biggest cause of neck pain is aging. As the body ages, the spaces in the spine narrow down and lead to increased pain in the neck area. Age also makes the muscles and ligaments of the neck become stiffer and weaker, which increases the chances of injury from moving the head too fast. Weight gain and maintaining a poor posture over the years only aid in worsening the pain.

The good news is that neck pain can be treated with the help of physical therapy using resistance bands. Combining bands with corrective exercises and stretches aims to improve functions of the neck as well as relieve pain. A case study held in Finland discovered that people who used resistance bands to decrease neck pain were four times more successful than the ones doing similar stretching exercises without the use of a band.

Jari Ylinen is a medical doctor who made more in-depth observations on how resistance band exercises eased chronic neck pain. Ylinen took 180 volunteers of different ages, all suffering from chronic neck pain. The volunteers were split into three different groups. The first group would just do simple neck stretching exercises without any added resistance. The second group added resistance bands to the same exercises. The third group, however, was required to avoid any exercises or stretches that included the strengthening of the neck area and were only given a basic workout routine to follow.

The two active groups also added lifting light free weights 2 out of 7 days a week. The exercise using free weights was aimed at working out their chest, shoulders, and arms. After one year, all three groups came back with different results when it came to chronic neck pain improvement.

The group that did no neck strengthening exercises but proceeded to follow a light workout regime had an improved neck movement of 10% and ease of rotation of 10%. Those working out without resistance bands but still doing neck strengthening exercises had a 28% improvement in neck movement and a 29% improvement in neck rotation.

On the other hand, the results of patients that used resistance bands were on a whole other level. Over a year, the group's neck movement had improved by 110% while the ease of rotatability was 80%. Here are some of these exercises you can practice in the comfort of your own home:

Cervical Extension Stretch

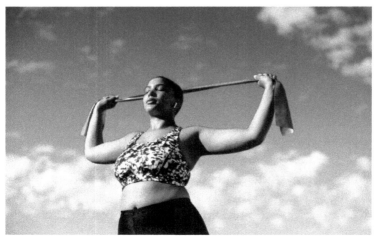

1. Keep the body in a vertical position
2. Place a thera resistance band at the back of your head
3. Grab the ends of the band with your hands and pull them slowly forward

4. During the exercise, keep the elbows in a 90° position and keep your head as straight as possible and your chin tucked and stiff
5. Maintain this position for 10 seconds and then rest
6. Repeat 3-5 times

Cross Cervical Extension Stretch

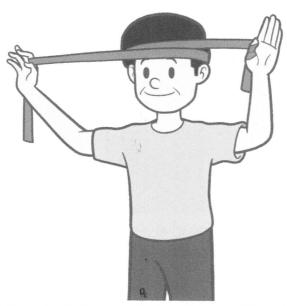

1. While maintaining a vertical position and keeping the thera band at the back of your head, cross the band over your forehead.
2. The only difference this time is that you will grab and pull the left end of the band with your right hand and the right end of the band with your left hand.
3. Keep elbows on the side in a 90° position while keeping your head straight and chin slightly tucked
4. Slowly pull one side of the band slowly outward before proceeding the same way with the other side
5. Maintain this position for 10 seconds and then rest
6. Repeat 3-5 times for each arm

Side Cervical Extension Stretch

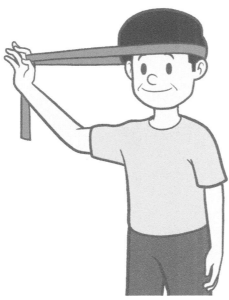

1. Maintain vertical position while wrapping your head with the loop band and grabbing both ends of the band with one hand.

2. Keep the elbow on the side in a 90° position while keeping your head straight and chin slightly tucked

3. Slowly pull the band outward until the elbow reaches a 120° position.

4. Maintain this position for 10 seconds and then rest before practicing the same stretch with the other hand.

5. Repeat 3-5 times for each arm

Keep in mind that not all people are the same. In rare cases, progressing neck pain might be a sign of an underlying condition that needs medical assistance. Make sure to contact your healthcare provider if your neck pain is accompanied by numbness, loss of coordination in the upper arm area, feeling nauseous, dizzy, unwell, extremely stiff, experiencing fever chills, or if the pain keeps getting worse even after taking over the counter medication.

Another common upper body pain is shoulder pain. Unlike any other part of the body, the shoulders are the biggest and most movable joint in our body. They are created by a group of four muscles working together with the help of tendons. The muscles and the tendons as a whole form what is known as the rotator cuff which makes the shoulder one of the most flexible parts of the body.

The most common reason for shoulder pain is due to the tendons getting stuck under the bone area. This occurs from bad posture over the years, or due to disuse of the muscles for a long time. There are many other reasons that cause the rotator cuff to become damaged or inflamed, which eventually leads to pain.

People who suffer from Bursitis, which is a condition that causes the fluid-filled sack of the shoulder to become inflamed. This sack is responsible for the smooth and flexible movement of the joints in the shoulder. So, when experiencing such inflammation, the shoulder area starts experiencing pain.

Lack of physical activity over the years could also cause what is known as the frozen shoulder. This is where the muscles and tendons become weak and lose mobility, causing pain whenever moving the shoulder. There are times when such pain might even come from another upper body part such as the neck.

People that suffer from chronic neck pain often experience some level of shoulder pain. However, this pain is often present only when sitting or lying down and not when moving the muscles.

Unlike neck pain, shoulder pain is a bit more complicated to ease. This is because there are different causes of shoulder pain which require different stretching exercises. Shoulders are more delicate and often require the assistance of a physical therapist to complete the exercise.

Thera bands with light resistance are often the best solution for easing shoulder pain for beginners. They add just the right resistance level to the muscles and prevent the risk of injury. The following are three corrective shoulder stretches you can do at home:

Reverse fly

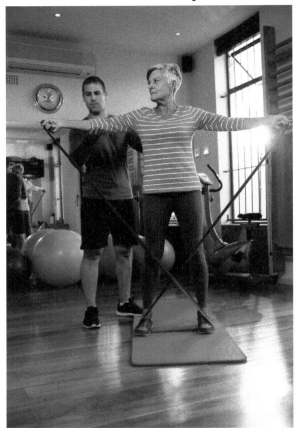

1. Place a thera band on the floor and stand in the middle of the band while keeping your feet shoulder-width apart
2. Cross the ends of the bands by grabbing the right end of it with your left hand and the left end of the band with your right hand
3. Slightly bend your knees and your upper body while making sure that you keep your spine in a relaxed and neutral position.
4. Pull the band outward at chest height with your palms facing down and elbows at 90°
5. Maintain the position for a couple of seconds before slowly returning back to the resting position
6. Repeat the stretch 5-10 times

Lateral raise

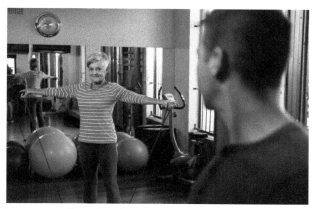

1. Continue standing in the middle of the band with legs open at shoulder-width
2. Straighten your body at a vertical position
3. Grab each end of the loop band with its corresponding hand
4. Keep your arms fully stretched at hip level
5. Pull the band upward by raising your arms to the side at shoulder height
6. Maintain the position for 3 seconds before slowly returning to the resting position
7. Repeat the stretch 5-10 times

Overhead band pull-apart

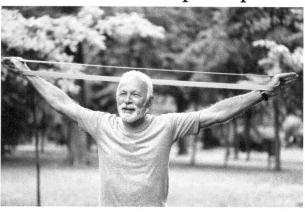

1. Grab your resistance band by both ends and hold it above your head
2. Keep your arms raised in a "Y" position
3. Pull the band outwards while slightly lowering your arms in the process
4. During the stretch keep your head and back straight to keep the shoulder blades down
5. Hold this position for approximately 3 seconds
6. Repeat 5-10 times

Tube bands can also be effective in easing shoulder pain. Sometimes, shoulder pain can be life-threatening. So, knowing when to call a doctor will, in some cases, even save your life. When experiencing sudden shoulder pain on your left side of your body that feels like a crushing sensation or if the pain spreads to your left jaw, arm, neck, or chest, make sure to call 911 and chew on aspirin with little to no water as these are signs of a heart attack.

Other times where you need to seek a healthcare provider is if shoulder pain is accompanied by swelling, redness, or pale bluish color on the shoulder and also if the pain becomes too severe it completely blocks the shoulder from moving.

Chronic arm pain on the other hand is an entirely different story! In fact, arm pain as you age all depends on how much you used them throughout your life. For example, people that have worked in a desk job writing all day will experience a lot more arm complications as they grow older. Unlike most parts of the body, the arms and legs do most of the moving. So, logically, having a good amount of muscle in these areas is crucial for mobility.

If these muscles are rarely put to use, then they will start weakening and shrinking. But, it isn't exactly the lack of muscle that causes pain in the arms. It's due to the injuries that come as a result of weakened muscles that make arms hurt. Arthritis is the most common reason why seniors experience chronic arm pain. The degrading of the joints in the arms leads to swelling and stiffness.

The good news is that healing arm pain does not need as much caution as shoulder pain does. In most cases, the pain goes away by itself in time. However, to heal the injuries that cause such pain you can always practice these corrective arm stretches.

Bow and Arrow

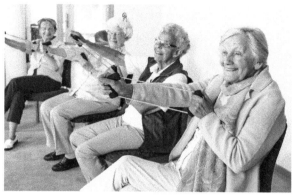

1. Sit on a chair and grab your resistance band by both ends
2. Hold one arm straight in front of your face at a 120° and the other one in front of your chest like you are about to pull an arrow
3. Imagine if the loop band is a bow and pull on it while keeping the straight arm in a stiff position
4. Maintain the position for 5-10 seconds
5. Repeat the stretch 3-5 times for each arm

Bicep Curl

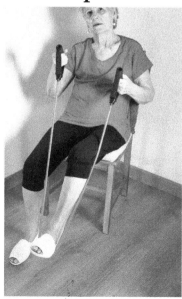

1. As you sit on a chair, place the tube or thera band on the floor and step in the middle of it
2. Grab each end of the loop band with its corresponding hand
3. Pull the band while keeping your palms facing up and your elbows at a 90° angle
4. Take turns pulling the band with each hand separately
5. Gently go to starting position as soon as you finish a full bicep curl
6. Repeat the stretch 8 times for each arm

Overhead triceps extension

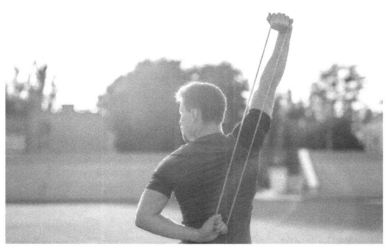

1. Stand in a vertical position
2. Wrap one end of your loop band with one hand while keeping your elbow at a 90° angle and place the hand behind your head
3. Put your other hand behind your back and grab the other end of the band
4. Pull the band with the arm placed behind your back until the arm is almost straight (Reminder: DO NOT straighten the arm fully as it increases the chances of injury)
5. Gently go to starting position as soon as you finish a full stretch
6. Repeat the stretch 5 times for each arm

And last but not least is back pain, which is the most common chronic pain among humans. According to statistics, back pain is one of the main reasons people end up seeing a doctor, miss important events, or even skip work. Chronic back pain can happen to adults of all ages, but unfortunately, it worsens with age. As the body gets older, the spinal structure and joints located in the back get damaged. This causes burning and exhausting pain throughout the entirety of the lumbar area of the spine.

One of the most common age-related conditions that cause back pain is degenerative arthritis, also known as arthritis of the spine. As the body ages, the cartilage that is present in the facet joint of the spine gets broken down. The breakdown of this cartilage starts as early as 15 years of age and never stops.

However, the amount that is broken down differs from person to person, as studies show that healthier people who work out regularly have a much slower breakdown process. Genetics also plays a significant role in developing degenerative arthritis.

86% of adults over the age of 60 suffer from this condition. Arthritis of the spine usually causes the most back pain during the morning and night, which can cause trouble sleeping. People suffering from the condition also experience intermittent aching of the back throughout the day or experience loss of mobility and stiffness of the back.

If left untreated, back pain can become fatal and affect the sciatic nerve located on the leg. Depending on how much the nerve is irritated, the symptoms can be as extreme as feeling massive pain when moving or walking. In some individuals, the pain becomes so severe it leads to temporary loss of mobility.

Because back pain is extremely common, it is not preventable. However, stopping the pain from progressing and also easing pain to some extent is possible with the proper rehabilitation exercises. Adding resistance to the back muscles increases strength in the lower back area. The stretches mentioned down below increase flexibility, ease the pain, and overall improve the quality of life.

Single Arm Stretch

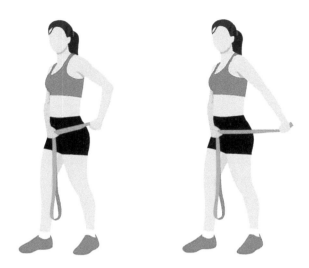

1. Stand in a vertical position and place one leg slightly forward
2. Take a short thera band or tube band and place grab it at both ends
3. Put your right hand on your left thigh or your left hand on your right thigh
4. Pull your left hand sideways while maintaining the elbow at a 90° angle
5. Hold the position for 2 seconds and bring the arm back to the resting position
6. Repeat 8 times for each arm

Seated Row

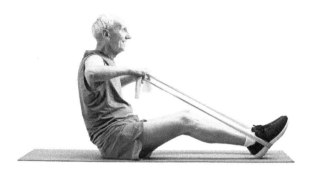

1. Sit on the ground (preferably on a yoga matt) and place a loop band around the feet
2. Make sure to wear athletic shoes and use a flat loop band with a low resistance to prevent injury
3. Grab each end of the band with the corresponding hand
4. Keep elbow at 90° angle at all times during the stretch
5. Pull the band until your hands reach your core/chest area
6. Hold the position for 2 seconds before slowly going back to starting position
7. Repeat the stretch 10 times

Cat/Cow Stretch

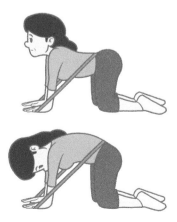

1. Place a long loop resistance band over your lower back and wrap each end of the band with the corresponding hand
2. Put both hands and knees on the ground while keeping your back relaxed
3. Inhale deeply before starting the stretch
4. Round your spine and tighten your belly in an upward curl position as you exhale
5. Then proceed to inhale and arch your spine while letting your belly loose
6. Repeat this stretch 8 times

It is important to keep in mind to call a medical professional if back pain gets worse even after taking over-the-counter medication. You should also call a doctor if you experience back pain along with unexplained weight loss, fever, or problems with bowel movements and urination.

Chapter 3: Rehab: Lower Body Pain:

Statistics show that by 2030, more than 25% of the U.S population will be aged 65 or older. Europe will also be experiencing similar growing numbers of seniors over the next decade. Although there are many causes why there is an increase in the elderly population, two of the most dominant ones are the decline in birth rates and most importantly the fact that life expectancy has increased.

The cause of higher life expectancy isn't because of healthcare and medicine evolving more than how both generation z and boomers managed their health. A study conducted by Blue Cross Blue Shield came to an interesting conclusion where researchers discovered that the younger generation had a much higher mortality rate than the older generation. This comes from a series of different factors.

One of the main reasons why generation z and boomers will live healthier and longer lives are due to their lifestyle. Having had a better work-life balance, active social life, and being less exposed to tempting processed food led these two generations to have lower rates of psychotic conditions, type 2 diabetes, severe depression, and endocrine conditions.

According to statistics, adults 60 and older are highly interested in gaining as much knowledge in maintaining their health further. They are more prone to watching what type of food they consume, learn about how their body and its functions, and are more concerned about their physical health. But despite living in better health conditions than the newer generations, chronic pain is inevitable among the older adult population.

More than half of the entire population over 60 years of age have experienced some sort of chronic pain, stiffness, and muscle weakness. This number only gets worse with 80% of the population over 70 years old having taken some sort of pain-killing medication throughout their senior years.

Chronic body pain generates over 100 billion dollars a year as it is one of the worst public health issues seniors face. Data indicated that almost half of patients who were experiencing body pain had worsened symptoms 6 months later. The cause of all this pain is linked to a condition that affects one in four older adults called chronic musculoskeletal pain or CMP.

CMP affects both the upper and lower body but affects the hip and knee area more severely. A study on the elderly living in retirement homes found that 90% of them had suffered from chronic lower body pain throughout their senior years. However, out of this 90%, 41% of them claimed to have experienced worsened symptoms that even led to unbearable pain and loss of mobility. It was later found that the majority of the older adults suffering unbearable pain were due to having CPM. The main cause of CPM progression is strongly linked to the disuse of the body.

Unfortunately, this condition has no cure, but seniors that started physical therapy and then continued to exercise had massive results when it came to pain relief and gaining more mobility. Starting off with light stretches using thera resistance bands and progressing by adding more workouts is proven to be the most effective way to prevent CMP from taking charge of your body. Three of the most chronic lower body pain people suffer from are hip, knees, and feet.

Hips are known for being more durable when it comes to pain and stiffness. This is mostly caused by the way it is built. The hip has the body's largest joint, and since it's bigger, it allows for more fluid movement.

But aging is far more powerful than any part of our body, no matter how durable it is. With that being said, even hips get damaged with age. Aging leads the cartilage existing in the joints of the hips to become more damaged. The muscles eventually lose their strength and bones become fragile. One thing leads to another up until the point where hips can become a threat to life.

A shocking number of senior deaths occur because of the hips. In fact, one-third of seniors that suffer a hip fracture pass away within 12 months of the injury. Older adults that have weak hips are five times more likely to die because of hip fractures than ones that have healthier hips. Although being a more durable part of the body, once damaged, hips will significantly reduce the quality of life, causing ongoing and unbearable pain accompanied by loss of mobility.

Osteoporosis is the lead factor that causes weakness of the hip and increases the chances of fracture. But as mentioned in chapter one, osteoporosis is manageable by stimulating and gaining bone mass by following a resistance band stretching workout routine. Apart from hip fractures, older people also develop sore hips which are caused by a couple of different age-related conditions.

People suffering from rheumatoid arthritis have the highest chances of hip pain. Rheumatoid arthritis causes inflammation of the hip joint and eventually leads to worsening pain if left untreated. The condition is oftentimes followed by loss of range of motion and stiffness of the hips. There are also cases where people have developed a limp from ongoing and untreated hip pain.

Unsuspected movement of the hip can also cause muscle strains or tendon strains. This leads them to become inflamed and prevents the hip from moving as it used to. The good news is that hip complications caused by muscle or tendon strains can easily be fixable by following simple stretches that heal and tighten hip muscles.

Hip pain is often associated with a set of different symptoms such as discomfort in areas of the joint, thigh, buttocks, and groin. If you want to prevent hip pain altogether before it occurs then staying active will reduce the risk of experiencing such complications as you age. However, if you are experiencing hip pain, a careful rehabilitation process is a must to overcome it.

One thing that is important to keep in mind is that exercising while experiencing hip pain is dangerous and even life-threatening. The only way to recover your hip is by corrective stretching of the hip with the help of loop resistance bands. Some stretching exercises you can practice are:

Clam Shells

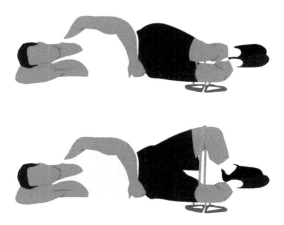

1. Place your legs inside a short loop band and lift the band slightly above the knee
2. Lie on your side with knees and hips slightly bent
3. Slowly open your thighs while keeping your heels together
4. Gently go to starting position as soon as you finish the stretch
5. When switching sides, AVOID using your back. Instead, use your upper body weight to reduce the risk of injury
6. Repeat the stretch 10-15 times on each side

Hip Abduction

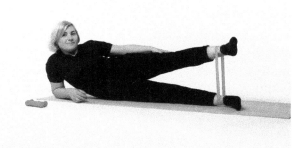

1. Place the short loop band a few inches under the knee while continuing to lie on the side
2. Straighten your legs and hips while placing your elbow on the ground to support your upper body
3. Pull the band upward with the leg that isn't touching the ground
4. Slowly come down to resting position
5. Repeat 8 times on each leg

Hip Bridges

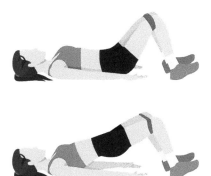

1. Place the short loop band around the knees
2. Lie in a flat in a relaxed position on the ground
3. Bend your knees halfway and keep them at shoulder-width
4. Then slowly lift your rear and gently come down again
5. Repeat the stretch 15 times

While performing regular daily stretches to heal hip pain, additional methods to ease the pain is by applying an ice pack to the hip area for a couple of minutes. Repeat this a couple of times a day to reduce inflammation until you start feeling better. If you are not a fan of cold icy packs touching your body then you can heat the painful area for a couple of minutes several times a day.

Another tip that helps a lot in the healing process is taking a warm shower before starting the corrective stretches. This will warm up the muscles and open up the arteries for better blood flow which will lessen the pain while stretching.

If the pain gets worse while performing stretches, feel a sudden blocking sensation around your hips, or experience sudden sharp pain, stop immediately and seek help from a healthcare provider. There are a handful of cases where people that have developed hip pain were unaware that their hip was fractured. In fact, it's best recommended to see a doctor as soon as hip pain occurs and get advice from a medical professional on the best road to recovery.

Knee pain is another common chronic pain that affects older adults. The pain can develop in different forms, with the most common ones being due to sudden injury or damaged cartilage of the joints. Your weight can also play a tremendous role in the development of knee pain. People who are overweight have a far greater risk of developing this kind of pain.

Being overweight exhausts the joints of the knees. The added pressure of the extra weight eventually starts damaging the knee joints up to the point where every step you take will become more challenging.

The truth is that your joints can hold up to four times your body weight until they collapse. So, for example, if your ideal weight is around 150 pounds (11.7 stone), your knees can hold up to 600 pounds (42.8 stone) before collapsing. That is why most morbidly obese people weighing 400 pounds or more start losing their mobility when they start reaching that weight. With every 10 pounds gained, the pressure that the knee joints hold is an additional 40 pounds more.

The bright side is that knee pain can be taken care of by following just a few simple tips and stretches. If you are in the starting phases of developing knee pain, lower the amount of exercise and focus more on stretching workouts with a loop resistance band. Try wearing running shoes that have good cushioning and that fit comfortably during your stretches as they will better support the knees and prevent them from experiencing too much-added pressure.

Seated Knee Extension

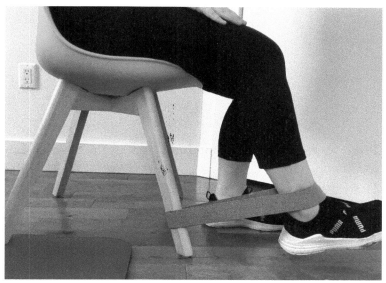

1. Sit on a chair and place a short loop band around one of the front legs of the chair
2. Put one leg inside the loop band at ankle level
3. Pull the band with your leg until it's slightly straightened
4. Hold the position for 3 seconds
5. Repeat 3-5 times for each leg

Crab Walk with Resistance Band

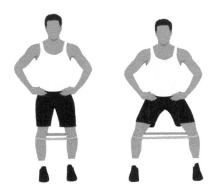

1. Place your legs inside a loop band and lift the band slightly above the knee
2. Hold a vertical posture with slightly bent knees and back while keeping your hands on your hips
3. Gently move one step sideways to open the legs even wider
4. Follow along with the other leg to narrow down the gap between the legs (Reminder: DO NOT close the legs fully for this stretch)
5. Do the stretch 8 times for each leg

Standing Leg Side Raises

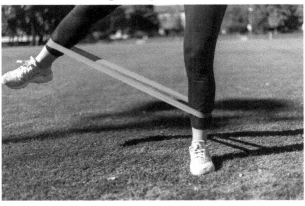

1. Place a short loop band around your ankles
2. Make sure to hold on to something, like a chair for balance
3. Keep your hips and shoulders facing slightly forward
4. Slowly pull the band sideways with your ankle while keeping your other leg slightly bent
5. Hold the position for 3 seconds before gently coming back to the resting position
6. Repeat 5 times for each leg

You can also ease knee pain by applying ice or heat in the painful area a few times a day. Never treat knee pain by yourself if the pain is caused by a recent injury. Also, it is best to call a medical professional if the knee pain on your knee continues even after you treat it at home for three days. If you have pain even when the knee is resting, your knee is deformed, makes a clicking noise when walking, becomes a red color, or doesn't open all the way out then it's best to see a doctor.

On the other hand, chronic ankle pain is caused by completely different factors. In most cases, you can predict if you are going to suffer from weak ankles as you age. This is because ankle pain is caused by how many times the ankle has been injured throughout your whole life. A percentage of the population sprain or injure their ankle a few times during their life. This causes the muscles and ligaments of the ankles to get damaged. In some cases, if the ankle doesn't get proper treatment after an injury, it can get permanently damaged.

Of course, the damage is not enough to leave an adult disabled, however, it does come to haunt you as you get older with chronic ankle instability or CAI. The condition affects 20% of people that have severely sprained or injured their ankle at some point in their lives. CAI causes the ankle to randomly roll to the side or become wobbly which increases the chances of an ankle injury and falls. CAI can be treatable by taking prescribed medication and corrective ankle stretches.

Another reason that causes ankle pain might be the fact that you are not wearing the right type of footwear. Wearing shoes that are too narrow, heavy, flat, or tight can cause many complications for the ankle. Investing in at least two pairs of shoes with supportive foam and a shock-absorbing midsole will make a huge difference.

Around 33% of adults 65 or older develop diabetes. Almost half of them suffer from diabetic peripheral neuropathy, which is a nerve complication that causes ongoing pain in the ankles. The condition also makes you lose some sense of coordination which increases the chances of falling and spraining the ankle.

The good news is that consistent ankle stretches with resistance bands will strengthen the muscles and bones of the ankles. The stretches will reduce pain and lower the chances of injury caused by weak ankles. The following includes three ways to heal damaged ankles.

Ankle Plantarflexion

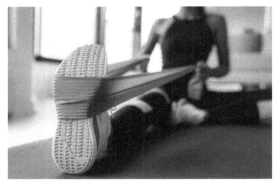

1. Place a loop resistance band around your foot.
2. Grab the ends of the band with both hands.
3. Pull the band towards the body and let your ankle slowly raise and your hamstrings. stretch.
4. Repeat 8 times on each ankle.

Inward Ankle Rotation

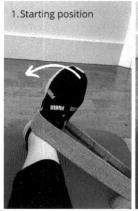
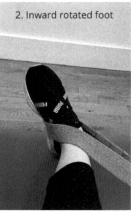

1. Tie one end of a loop band to the leg of a table or bed.

2. Sit on a yoga mat and open your legs.

3. Move your foot inward in a circular motion while keeping the heel touching the ground at all times (Reminder: the stretch will NOT be effective if you pull the entire foot inward. Focus on moving the ankle rather than any other part of the foot).

4. Gently go to the starting position as soon as you finish a full stretch.

5. Repeat the stretch 8 times for each ankle.

Outward Ankle Rotation

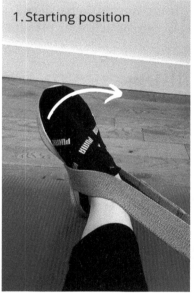

1. Starting position

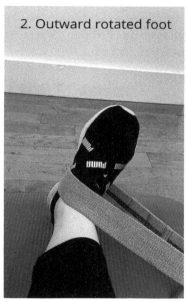

2. Outward rotated foot

1. For the outward rotation keep the same position as the inward rotation stretch.

2. Move your foot outward without moving the heel.

3. Also, repeat this stretch 8 times for each ankle.

If the pain doesn't get better within the first three days of practicing the stretches or if your ankle hurts even more while doing the movement with the band, it is best to talk to go see your doctor. You should also call a doctor if your ankle gets swollen for more than a few days, and turns bluish, red, or purple. Such signs indicate that your ankle might have experienced some kind of injury, or are symptoms of diabetes.

NOTE: DO NOT practice any of the mentioned ankle exercises if you have recently sprained your ankle and it has swollen. Instead, apply only ice (no heat) on the swollen area and get the ankle checked at a medical center.

And last but not least, is the most complex part of the body; the foot. It is made up of 26 bones and 33 joints working together with the help of over 120 pieces of individual muscles, tendons, and nerves. The foot's complexity allows it to bear your whole body weight, keep balance while walking, and is responsible for shock absorption.

But as you age, the feet get "worn out" and eventually become prone to numerous problems. In time, the sole also starts wearing down. It becomes wider and flatter, which causes pain when walking. Foot pain is caused by living a sedentary lifestyle, using unsupportive shoes, wearing heels, or obesity. Follow these essential foot stretches to prevent further foot problems and ease the pain:

Foot Pull-Ups

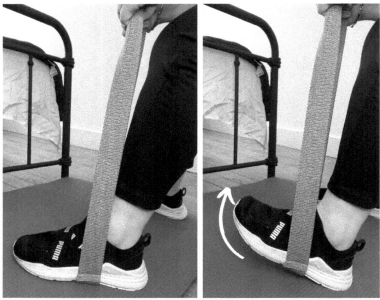

1. Secure a loop band under one foot by wrapping it around two or three times.
2. Make sure the loop band stays in the middle of the heel and toes of the foot.

3. Grab the band with both hands tight and firm.

4. Keep the heel of the foot you are stretching on the floor while slowly raising the front part. up.

5. Repeat the stretch 15 times with two sets on the foot that causes pain.

Foot Push Downs

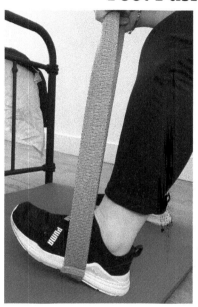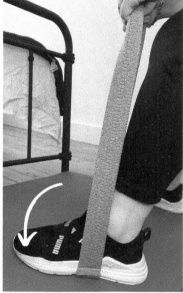

1. This stretch is almost identical to the foot push-ups. The only difference lies in the movement of the foot.

2. For the push downs, instead of raising the foot, you are going to aim at lowering the foot down.

3. This means that the starting position of this stretch will be keeping your heel on the floor and your foot upwards while slowly lowering it.

4. Repeat the stretch 15 times with two sets on the foot that causes pain.

Foot Turn Outs

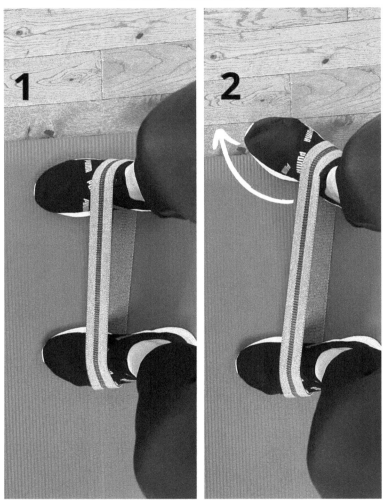

1. Continue keeping the band wrapped on the targeted foot and the remainder of the band hooked by your other foot
2. Pull the band to the side using the foot you are targeting
3. Make sure that the heel doesn't move and remains in contact with the ground at all times throughout the stretch
4. Repeat the stretch 15 times with two sets

Chapter 4: Resistance Bands and Yoga

You might be thinking, "I can't do yoga, I can't even reach my knees, let alone my toes!" Well, as shocking as this might seem, practicing yoga as an older adult doesn't have to turn you into one of those freaky circus acrobats. Many people are left with the impression that the main purpose of yoga is to make the body reach new limits in terms of flexibility. But the truth is, that's not the case. The lack of flexibility you have in yoga is your greatest advantage!

The truth is that being too flexible or hypermobile can be a bad thing when practicing yoga. Hypermobility is more frequent in young adults and rare in adults over 60. But according to plenty of yoga instructors, being able to naturally reach your feet and do a full leg split effortlessly leads to looseness of the joints that causes hypermobile people to develop pain and even cause injury as they get older.

Yoga is not about reaching new records of flexibility. It's more about breathing techniques, muscle strengthening, and corrective stretches for improved motion, stability, and prevention of chronic pain. People who practice yoga with resistance bands have revealed that they experience a feeling of "being held together" and increase muscle strength.

The reason yoga is more beneficial using resistance bands is that it slows down the movement of the exercise from the added resistance when you pull. This allows you to increase muscle mass rather than going too far with the stretches. Going overboard with stretches can also harm tendons and lead to injury. That is why it's important to keep in mind the main purpose when doing yoga exercises, which is to gain strength and improve the overall quality of life and not to reach new limits when stretching.

Yoga has been practiced by human civilization for more than 5000 years. It was first practiced in Northern India and was strongly linked to religion. Indians used yoga as a way to connect with a higher power and increase awareness. In modern days, yoga is a globally widespread practice. It is commonly used among all ages as it is proven to be both physically and mentally beneficial. Older adults who practice yoga were less stressed, had better sleep, and were more physically flexible when compared to adults who didn't include it in their daily life.

According to statistics, the number of Americans over the age of 50 that practiced yoga rose from 4 million in 2012 to more than 14 million in 2016. That is almost 4 times higher. The growth in popularity isn't just a coincidence. The reason yoga practice has reached an all-time high is that people are now starting to realize that the benefits of yoga are more than what was expected.

Another reason why yoga is a great choice for seniors is that it holds a lesser risk of getting injured. Using resistance bands solely for building up muscle takes some time and patience to adapt. Plus, it can be dangerous for beginners. That is why it is recommended to start using resistance bands to first heal the body through rehabilitation exercises, and then slowly start combining it with yoga.

This will gradually help the body heal at its maximum capacity which will allow it to regain double the strength it could have regained by immediately starting to do strengthening exercises. Another thing about yoga is that it is never too late to start, no matter how old you get! (Just make sure to get a doctor's approval before you start including it in your routine.)

Yoga has many life-changing health benefits. One of the benefits older adults like the most about practicing yoga is that it relieves and keeps chronic pain away. The previous chapters informed you on how you can relieve chronic pain. But aging will always do its thing and bring this pain back if you go back to your usual routine. Yoga prevents that. This is because it alleviates the areas where the pain is present.

A study found something unique and new about how chronic pain is connected to stress. The study found that although the pain was due to complications that came with aging, it was highly impacted by the levels of stress a person experienced in their lives.

The area of the body that caused the pain was more inflamed in seniors that had a more stressful life than the ones who didn't. And because yoga has a huge impact on fighting stress levels, it automatically helps reduce inflammation in the painful areas of the body. Typically, statistics show that seniors that start practicing yoga consistently, require less pain medication after around the fourth week.

Yoga also helps with insomnia. Up to 48% of adults over the age of 60 have experienced insomnia symptoms. While 12%-20% of adults suffer from regular insomnia disorder. Surprisingly, yoga has shown to be more effective in soothing levels of insomnia than drinking herbal sleep tea.

There have even been instances that it has been more effective than sleep medication. This is all due to the impact yoga has on your breathing. By practicing your breathing technique with yoga exercises, your breathing automatically slows down. When this happens, your body produces more melatonin, which is a sleep-inducing hormone that is often lacking in adults who experience insomnia symptoms.

The Centers for Disease Control and Prevention highly recommend seniors practice yoga to fight high blood pressure. Also known as "the silent killer" high blood pressure is common in half of the people over the age of 55. But the thing is that many adults are not even aware of having this problem. This is all because in most cases, high blood pressure does not cause any signs of symptoms or illness.

Its effects come suddenly and instantly, usually with a stroke, sudden kidney disease or heart disease, and even vascular dementia. If lifestyle changes are not made to decrease blood pressure then its sudden effects may end up reducing the quality of life. Many seniors have reported having lower blood pressure after their very first day of doing yoga.

The biggest thing that is often overlooked by seniors is stress. Not managing stress levels can cause severe changes to your body. Stress is universally known for speeding up the aging process, making you look older. Seniors that do not manage stress or experience more stress in life experience what is called an internal fight or flight response. When you experience constant high levels of stress your autonomic and endocrine systems in the body will be activated. This leads your body to respond in unregulated ways, which is known as the fight or flight response.

Although it varies from person to person, seniors have a more hidden response to stress than younger adults do. Usually, younger adults respond to stress by lashing out, screaming, shutting down, and avoiding. Seniors on the other hand respond to stress by experiencing frequent headaches, increased blood pressure, shortness of breath, and increased blood sugar just to name a few. Seniors that suffer from dementia also experience high-stress levels that are mostly created by confusion.

Practicing yoga lets you focus more on your breathing which allows more oxygen to enter the bloodstream. As the oxygen levels in your body increase, your heart relaxes and your heartbeat slows down. Higher levels of oxygen in the bloodstream also help in relaxing the tension in the abdomen area where stress pain is usually felt. Focusing on our breathing is also a great way to be in the present moment and practice mindfulness.

Yoga prevents falls and injury. Because yoga is also a muscle strengthening practice, it leads to better stability and balance. It is highly known for strengthening the back muscles and core muscles, which is the primary reason why it can help you with better balance and prevent falls.

Holding a yoga pose for several breaths is a highly efficient way to improve body flexibility. This is because it allows the connective tissues and the muscles to relax. The relaxation of the muscles causes them to loosen up and give you the benefit of increasing your body's range of motion.

Yoga also improves respiration. Lungs do not have any muscle. However, you can still strengthen your lungs to hold more oxygen by practicing yoga. Your lungs fully mature at the age of 25. But, after the age of 35 lungs start deteriorating. This explains why you may experience shortness of breath more frequently as you age. Even though lung deterioration cannot be prevented, it can be slowed down as a process.

What happens as you age is that the Alveoli of the lungs lose their shape through time, which causes them to become baggy. The diaphragm also plays a huge role in shortness of breath. Aging weakens the diaphragm, which causes difficulty when inhaling and exhaling. One study found that women that followed a 3-month yoga program had less trouble breathing and falling short of breath.

Even though yoga offers some amazing benefits for the mind and body, it is always a good idea to talk to your healthcare provider and get professional recommendations before starting yoga. Some adults may not be capable of accomplishing a certain set of yoga exercises due to their medical conditions.

For example, people that suffer from glaucoma, which is an eye condition caused by damage to the optic nerve, should not practice any sort of yoga exercise with their head down. This is because too much blood to the head can increase eye pressure and further damage the optic nerve. Your doctor will give you similar advice if you suffer from any complications or conditions.

The next step to prepare for yoga is to gather all of the gear that is necessary to start your exercises. The first and most important thing to keep in mind before starting any yoga session is to wear loose clothing. Because yoga is tightly connected to breathing exercises, wearing tight clothing can cause unease. It can also impact the effectiveness of the practice as wearing tight clothing doesn't allow your body to fully inhale, leading to lower levels of stress being reduced.

When it comes to shirts, it's best to find a stretchy, light, and fitted top.

You would not want anything too loose as the shirt can end up all in your eyes in case you bend down during a stretch. Legwear is the most complicated, as it might tighten the belly area. Finding legwear that is light on the belly and does not fall when exercised is as rare as gemstones. But it's not impossible to find them! Footwear on the other hand is not needed when practicing yoga as the practice is originally done barefoot. If you would prefer to wear something, then wearing a pair of non-slip socks will do the trick.

Yoga doesn't need any other gear besides the mat, and of course, the resistance bands. When doing more traditional yoga exercises, a yoga mat is crucial. When it comes to choosing a mat, you need one that is as long (if not a bit longer) than you are when you lie down. Also, the material of the mat depends on its price. Although price doesn't necessarily impact the quality of practicing yoga, it does indicate the kind of quality the mat is built from.

Cheap mats are made from PVC while the more expensive ones are made with materials such as cotton, rubber, or jute, which are more environmentally friendly. When choosing the thickness of the mat don't go with anything that is more than half an inch thicker. Thicker yoga mattresses can cause you to lose balance and get injured. Thick mats are also a huge pain when it comes to carrying them around as they are pretty heavy.

The last step to prepare for a yoga session is to always start slowly. Keep in mind that you need to get enough rest between each yoga exercise, especially if you are a beginner. Do not go to the next exercise immediately. Give your body 20-40 seconds to relax in between each exercise.

Also, yoga is not a competition. If you are doing yoga along with your friend, partner, or collectively, remember to do the stretch at your own pace. Practicing yoga is done by doing whatever makes you feel comfortable so you can focus on your breathing and mindfulness.

Another very important thing before starting yoga is knowing that it should never hurt. You might feel a slight burning sensation that comes from the resistance band pulls, but any intense burning or other body pain means that you are unnecessarily pushing yourself too far during the exercise. Whenever you feel that a certain yoga position is causing you pain or discomfort, then focus on other exercises that are easier to complete.

Since every yoga position requires you to also practice breathing techniques, it's important to know how to properly breathe during exercises. You need to first relax the abdomen before inhaling for 3-4 seconds. Do not force yourself to fill up your lungs with as much air as possible when inhaling. The right way to do it is to inhale normally, neither too fast nor too slow, but as much as you feel comfortable. Then immediately exhale slowly, for 6-8 seconds.

There are many types of yoga. All have different focuses. In the following practices, you will be learning some of the best yoga exercises from the easiest exercises to start with up to more traditional exercises. Preparing for yoga is the first step to ensuring that you are doing the practice right.

Here are some easy and highly effective yoga exercises you can start even if you have never practiced it before. The first pose you will want to start with does not include resistance bands. Look at it more as a warm-up and a preparation for the yoga session you are about to do. The exercise is called the tree pose and its main purpose is to strengthen your balance for the upcoming yoga positions. If you are exercising at home you can also use a chair or the wall when performing this position for the first time.

Tree pose

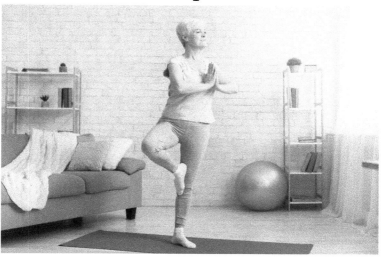

1. Stand up in a straight position
2. Straighten your back and open your chest for air to effortlessly fill your lungs.
3. Stand close to a chair or wall for stability
4. Raise your hands up straight above your head
5. Put one leg on the other leg's calf
6. Do a few breaths while holding the pose
7. Rest for 20-40 seconds before continuing with the other leg

If you find it difficult to maintain balance, then use one hand to hold on to a chair or a wall while continuing to keep the other hand up straight. As you get better at it, remove your hand from the chair or wall for a few seconds to further improve balance. Only do this if you are confident that you can maintain balance by yourself for a few seconds. If you are not confident enough, do not let go of the chair or wall while performing the exercise.

Upper body stretch

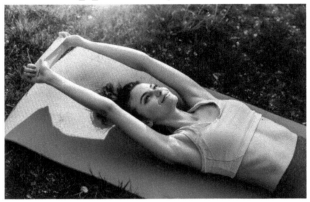

1. Lie down on a yoga mat
2. Hold a short loop band with both hands
3. Keep your back straight and relaxed
4. Keep both arms and legs stretched
5. Maintain position for several breaths

Side bends

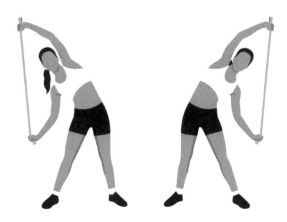

1. Take the thera band and place it above your head
2. Open feet hip-width and stand straight or sit on a chair
3. Keep body straight and relaxed
4. Slowly go down sideways while exhaling and come up inhaling
5. Repeat several times on both sides
6. Rest for 20-40 seconds before switching sides

Keep the head tight when doing the exercise and avoid moving it. Allow it to move along with your body. Make sure you are keeping your hands straight. The only thing that should be moving in this position is your spine. Now, when it comes to the breathing technique, inhale as soon as you bend down. Exhale while coming up in the starting position and inhale again while bending down. Repeat this cycle for a few breaths.

Chest stretch

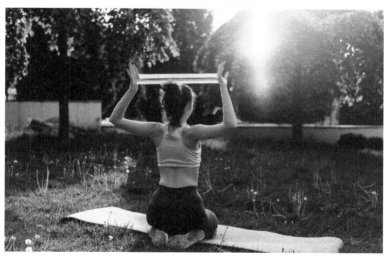

1. Maintain sitting position
2. Hold a thera band or loop band with both hands
3. Make sure your hands are behind your head
4. Keep the band slightly pulled while inhaling and exhaling
5. Maintain position for several breaths

Arm stretch

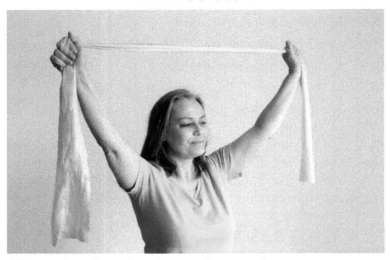

1. Place a short loop band around your wrists
2. Stand straight or sit down straight on a chair
3. Hold both hands in front of you and keep them straightened
4. Keep the band slightly pulled while inhaling and exhaling
5. Repeat for a few breaths until your arms feel fatigued

Close the yoga session by repeating the tree pose used you opened the session with. While holding on to a chair, try to practice the pose with your eyes closed this time. Focus deeply on your breathing and keep your mind in the present moment.

While doing this you can also focus on the feeling of your foot touching the calf, the feeling of your hand holding on to the chair, the outdoor noises, or indoor silence. This final closing practice not only helps with balance but also reduces stress levels, decreases blood pressure, and releases healthy amounts of melatonin hormones.

Chapter 5: Shoulder Exercises

Science has yet to find how to fully prevent the effects that come with age. But nature has given us a solution right in front of our doorsteps, which is the ability to exercise our body anytime and anywhere that we want to. It has always been one of the thousands of medicines that nature has provided us with. Yet, people still take exercising for granted and see it as a chore rather than a privilege that mankind is equipped with.

If you're a senior, you may want to consider strength training as an option for improving your health and fitness. The following chapters will help you determine whether strength training is right for you and how to get started.

Strength training has many benefits, including improved bone density, muscle mass, balance, posture, and lower-back strength. It can also help improve overall body composition by increasing lean muscle mass while decreasing body fat. This means that your body will burn more calories throughout the day—even when you're at rest.

Strength training is also known to reduce risk factors associated with osteoporosis (bone loss), type 2 diabetes, heart disease, high blood pressure, obesity, depression, and anxiety. By adding strength training to your weekly routine, you may be able to reduce or even reverse some of these risk factors in just a few months.

Strength training is one of the best things you can do for your health at any age. It's never too late to start. Studies show that people who start as late as age 60 will see health benefits from strength training. If you've been thinking about starting but haven't yet taken that first step yet, here are some reasons why now is a great time to get started.

In the United States, more than 50 percent of adults over the age of 65 are considered obese or overweight. Obesity increases the risk for type 2 diabetes, heart disease, and other chronic illnesses. Exercise is one of the best ways to maintain a healthy weight and improve your overall health.

It can even delay — or even prevent — many of these diseases from developing in the first place. If you're like most seniors, you've probably heard about how important exercise is for your overall health and well-being. However, many people find it hard to get motivated to start an exercise routine.

Exercising with resistance bands is considered an anaerobic exercise but bands can be dangerous if used improperly. Always use a piece of furniture nearby (like a strong chair or table) while doing exercises that involve standing on your hands or feet. This will give you something to instantly hold on to in case you lose balance.

Don't allow more than one person to hold each side of a resistance band at once unless it is specifically designed for multiple users (such as resistance tubes). You should also use caution with heavy resistance band levels (usually the darker colored bands). If you have fragile wrists or ankles, use caution when using heavy resistance bands because they may cause discomfort or even injure your wrists or ankles due to their extreme nature. Be aware of how much force is being exerted by each band and always be careful when using them. It is recommended to start with light bands and move up to medium level if you are an older adult.

Now, anaerobic exercises are slightly different from both rehab and yoga. Although both rehabilitation of the body and yoga practices are technically considered branches of exercise, they serve more for healing and stretching the body. Anaerobic exercise mostly focuses on gaining strength, and power, burning fat, and training the body to reach new limits.

Sure, all three types of physical activity are strongly tied to one another and have a lot of things in common. For example, all of them are vital for maintaining good mental health, reducing stiffness, and increasing muscle and bone mass and come with a long list of health benefits.

Another key difference between anaerobic exercise is that it does not focus on breathing techniques to gain energy. It involves more intense activities that do not last longer than 1 or 2 minutes. After fully healing from rehab training, and after practicing yoga for a few weeks, your body is likely capable of handling basic anaerobic exercises. It is always best to talk to a medical professional at first.

Weakening of the shoulders due to inactivity can lead to an increased risk of injury such as damage of the muscles and tendons of the rotator cuff. These injuries can happen to any age group, but they are most common in people over 40. A rotator cuff is a group of four muscles that allow you to raise and rotate your arm. It also helps keep the ball of your shoulder joint in its socket.

The most common injury to this area is a tear in the supraspinatus tendon, which passes through the middle of your shoulder and attaches to the top of your arm bone (humerus). The supraspinatus is one of the four muscles that make up the rotator cuff. As its name suggests, it helps lift your shoulder toward your ear and rotate it outward from your body (abduction).

Pain from this type of tear comes on gradually, often after lifting something heavy or repetitive movements such as throwing a ball or swinging a golf club for many years. It may feel like a burning sensation or stiffness when you raise your arm above shoulder level, but there's no swelling or bruising. If left severely untreated, some tears heal on their own with time and rest, but others need surgery to repair them.

Frozen shoulder is another painful condition that makes it difficult to move your shoulder. It occurs when the tissue around the joint becomes stiff and tight. This causes pain and limited motion of the affected shoulder.

There are several theories about how frozen shoulders happen. The most common theory is that it happens when surrounding tissue becomes scarred. This scar tissue then restricts movement in the joint and causes pain when you try to move your arm. Other theories include cartilage degeneration, nerve damage, and muscle imbalance or weakness at the joint.

Frozen shoulders can affect people of all ages, but it most often affects people between 40 and 60 years old. It's also more common in women than men (2:1 ratio). Individuals who have diabetes, thyroid disease, Parkinson's disease, or heart disease are at higher risk for developing frozen shoulders.

People who have had surgery on their shoulders are also more likely to develop this condition because they don't use their arms as much after surgery than before it happened. If you injured your shoulder during an accident or fall and haven't used it much since then, you may develop a frozen shoulder from lack of use over time.

Arthritis is the most common joint disease and affects more than 50 million people in the United States. Arthritis causes pain, stiffness, and swelling of the joints, and can lead to deformity and disability if not properly managed. Arthritis in the shoulder is called shoulder osteoarthritis. It is a type of degenerative arthritis that causes pain and swelling in one or both shoulders.

This condition starts as early as age 50, although it can begin at any age. The first symptom is increasing pain while lifting or rotating your arms. This pain is mostly felt at the shoulder area. You may also experience stiffness after sleeping on one side of your body. As osteoarthritis progresses, painful movement becomes more common, especially during activities that require overhead movements like throwing a ball or lifting heavy objects overhead (such as groceries).

The most common cause of osteoarthritis is overuse. Overuse occurs when your joints are used too much for too long with no rest periods to allow them to recover from injury or stress. A sudden injury may also lead to osteoarthritis if you continue using an injured joint too much before it has healed properly.

Balancing a yoga and strength training routine in your life is extremely crucial if you want to reduce or prevent any of these shoulder conditions. As mentioned previously, the shoulders are one of the largest areas of the body. Because they are the number one mobility provider for the upper body, weakened or damaged shoulders highly impact the quality of life. A great way to start a shoulder strengthening workout is by practicing good posture.

Wall press

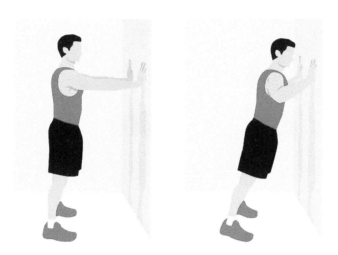

1. Stand up straight against a wall
2. Keep head, neck, shoulders, hip, and heels up against the wall
3. Keep your shoulders straight
4. Make sure your arms are straight and your palms are against the wall
5. Keep your feet closed
6. Keep the posture for 2 minutes while practicing deep breathing

This will straighten the shoulders as well as feed them with a good amount of oxygen to start the shoulder strengthening exercises.

Front raise

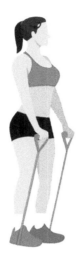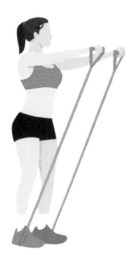

1. Step on a long loop or thera band with both feet
2. Grab the ends of the band with both hands
3. Keep your legs straight and open them shoulder-width
4. Keep shoulders and neck straight and firm
5. Place both hands in front of you at a 90° angle with palms facing down
6. Pull the band upward, fully straightening your arms above your head
7. Slowly go to starting position
8. Repeat 8 times with 3 sets

Lateral raises

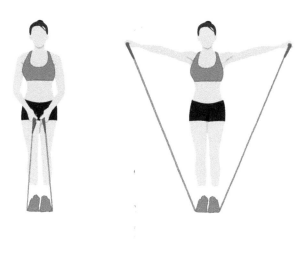

1. Maintain the same position of the front raise exercise
2. Bring your arms to the sides at a 90° angle while holding on to the band
3. Close your legs fully while continuing to keep them straight
4. Pull the thera band above your head in a "Y" position
5. Slowly come back down to starting position
6. Repeat 6-8 times with 3 sets

When doing this exercise, it is not necessary to fully stretch your arms above your head. Take it easy and pull the band over your head as far as you feel comfortable.

One-sided lateral raise

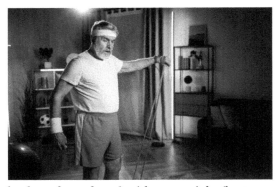

1. Step in the long loop band with your right foot
2. Grab the other end of the band with your right hand
3. Keep your hand straight and on the side with the palm facing down
4. Open legs at shoulder width and keep them straight
5. Keep shoulder and head straight while pulling the band sideways
6. Pull until it reaches shoulder height
7. Repeat 8 times on each side with 2 sets

The shrug pull

**SHOULDER
SHRUG**

WITH RESISTANCE BAND

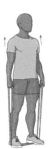 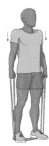

1. Step on a thera band with both feet
2. Keep your legs straight and open them shoulder-width
3. Wrap the ends of the band with both hands until the band is tight and stretched
4. Keep arms down and straight
5. Pull your shoulders up like you are shrugging
6. Lower the shoulders slowly in starting position
7. Repeat 8 times with 3 sets

Upright Row

UPRIGHT ROW

WITH RESISTANCE BAND

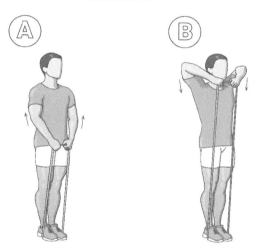

1. Step on a long loop band with both feet
2. Grab the ends of the band with both hands
3. Keep your legs straight and close
4. Put your hands in front of you at pelvic level
5. Pull the band upward until they reach the front of your chin
6. Slowly go to starting position
7. Repeat 8 times with 3 sets

Band dislocates

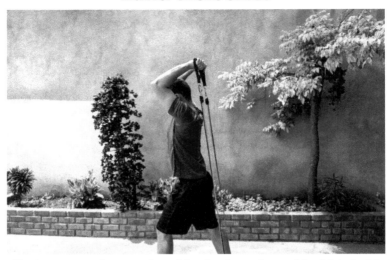

1. Grab your resistance band by both ends and hold it behind your back

2. Keep your arms in a 90° angle above your head

3. Pull the band upwards while slightly lifting your arms in the process

4. During the stretch keep your head and back straight to keep the shoulder blades down

5. Hold this position for approximately 3 seconds

6. Repeat 5-10 times

When you use resistance bands for weight training, the bands have the advantage of stimulating your shoulders just as if you are doing real-world work, such as lifting objects, but without all the dangers that come along with it.

Keep in mind that shoulder strengthening exercises are not recommended to practice if you have chronic or severe shoulder pain. To prevent injury or worsening a condition you may suffer from, you need to get a medical professional's opinion to safely start these shoulder exercises.

Chapter 6: Torso Exercises

The reason why this chapter is called torso and not abdominal exercises is that it's not just what is in front of your body that you need to strengthen, it's also what's around it. By definition, the torso is the trunk of your body. It includes your abdominal muscles, your side muscles, and your back muscles.

The core consists of three layers: anterior (front), lateral (side), and posterior (back). Each layer has its own set of muscles that work together to keep you balanced when standing upright or doing other activities such as walking or bending over to pick something up off the floor. The major muscle groups include:

Rectus abdominis: This is the muscle that makes up the bulk of what people see as a six-pack or a washboard stomach.

External obliques: These muscles run diagonally down each side of your abdomen and are used in side bending and twisting movements.

Internal obliques: Located beneath the external obliques on either side of your abdomen, these muscles assist with rotation and bending, such as when twisting to throw a pitch or swinging a golf club.

Transverse abdominis: This flat muscle sits beneath all other abdominal muscles and wraps around your entire torso like a corset from front to back. It helps stabilize your spine, especially during heavy lifting.

The core — sometimes called the "powerhouse" for its role in generating power and strength — is made up of a complex network of muscles and connective tissues that runs from the base of your skull to the top of your pelvis. This area includes your lower back, hips, abdomen, pelvic floor, and deep hip muscles. Your core is critical for good posture, balance, and movement. It also plays a role in breathing and digestion. Because the core covers such a large area of your body, it has its own chapter in this book. The benefits of strengthening your torso include:

Improved posture. A strong torso helps support the spine and maintain good alignment from head to toe. This reduces strain on ligaments, tendons, and other tissues that support the spine, as well as on joints throughout the body. Stronger abdominal muscles reduce lower back pain by improving posture and reducing back curvature. If you also want to avoid injuries like falling or tripping over objects, you need strong abdominal muscles to support your spine. Stronger spinal muscles will also help you lift heavier objects with greater ease, which reduces the strain on other parts of your body such as your arms and legs.

Better balance and coordination. Stronger muscles help you maintain balance when you're standing still or moving quickly; they also improve coordination between different muscle groups used in movement (such as walking or running). Whether you're lifting something heavy or bending over to tie your shoes, a strong torso will help you perform better in your daily activities.

Better athletic performance. Strengthening your torso also helps you perform better during sports that require quick bursts of energy such as tennis or golf (it can also help prevent injury during such sports). Stronger abdominals may help improve athletic performance by increasing power output from the legs during sprinting or jumping movements.

Relieved pain from sciatica and back injuries. A strong torso can help reduce pressure on nerves in the lower back caused by disc herniation or spinal stenosis (narrowing). This may relieve sciatica-type pain that shoots down the leg. A strong torso also helps stabilize the spine after surgery or injury, which may reduce pain and increase mobility during recovery.

More energy for everyday activities. Many of us spend our days sitting at desks or hunched over computers, which can lead to fatigue or back pain when we try to stand up straight again. By strengthening your core muscles, you'll feel more energized so that you can do everyday tasks without getting tired as fast!

You can strengthen your core through exercises such as planks and crunches. Planks are great exercises to strengthen the back and abdominal muscles. They also improve posture and balance, and they help prevent back pain. To do a plank, lie face down on the floor on your elbows and toes (make sure to wear shoes), holding yourself up in a straight line from head to heels.

Hold this position for as long as possible without letting your hips sag or your lower back arch. If you can't hold this position for 30 seconds, try holding it for 10 seconds at first and increase your time gradually over time until you're able to hold it for 30 seconds without allowing any sagging or arching in your back or hips. If this still seems like a challenge, then place both knees on the ground and continue to perform the plank. You can slowly upgrade to a regular plank once you feel more confident or after having gained more strength by exercising regularly.

Crunches help build abdominal strength by exercising the rectus abdominis muscle — the "six-pack" muscle that runs down the front of your abdomen — along with other muscles in your back and hips. While crunches are an effective way to strengthen these muscles, they don't necessarily improve overall function or mobility in daily life.

For example, if you have poor posture or weak hips or glutes (buttocks), then these imbalances may contribute to poor movement patterns that can lead to lower back pain over time. The best way to fix this is by adding resistance bands to your torso strengthening exercises. Here are a list of torso strengthening exercise you can perform:

Torso: Chest

Chest press

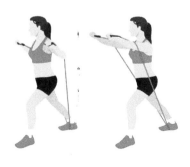

1. Step on a long loop band or tube band with one foot
2. Place the other foot forward and bend it slightly
3. Grab the other end of the loop band (the band should be behind you)
4. Pull by moving your arms in front of your chest
5. Go back to the starting position (arms should not go behind your back. Keep them parallel with your shoulders)
6. Repeat 6 times for each leg

Chest crossover

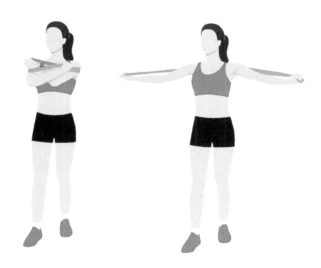

1. Place a thera band around your back
2. Grab each side of the band with its corresponding hand
3. Straighten your arms
4. Keep your back straight and your neck gently tucked
5. Cross your arms in front of your chest
6. Repeat for 8-10 reps

Torso: Upper Abdomen

Cobra stretch

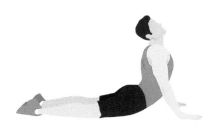

1. Lie face down on your yoga mat
2. Keep your legs straight
3. Slowly raise your body up while curing your back
4. Keep shoulders straight
5. Maintain the position for 20 seconds while breathing normally

Alternate heel touches

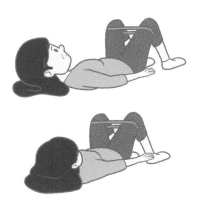

1. Lie down on the yoga mat
2. Keep legs bent with the sole on the ground
3. Keep arms straight

4. Slightly raise your head in a semi-crunch position
5. Move your core from the side
6. While moving pretend as if you are trying to reach your feet with your arms
7. Repeat for 10 reps

Torso: Mid-back muscles

Overhead pull

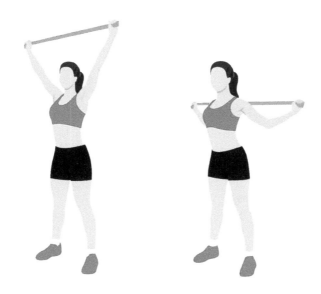

1. Stand in a vertical position
2. Grab a band on both sides with each hand
3. Position the band over your head
4. Pull the band outward while bringing it down to your back
5. Repeat for 6-8 reps

Chapter 7: Arm Exercises

The arms are an important part of the body and can be used as a gauge for overall fitness. If you have weak arms, there is a good chance that you will also have weak legs and a weak back. Strong arms allow you to keep yourself in good shape for years to come. A strong set of arms makes it possible for you to lift heavy items with ease, do more push-ups and pull-ups, throw objects farther, swing harder at golf, etc.

A lot of people think that you can only get healthy arms by lifting heavy weights. But the truth is, you can also get toned and shapely arms by working out using only resistance banks. Hands down, the best way to build strong, toned arms is strength training. When you work out your muscles, they get bigger and stronger to handle the stress of being used. As a result, they grow.

In addition to arm-related exercises, there are many other ways that you can strengthen your arms. For example, if you want to improve your grip strength or make it easier on yourself when lifting heavy items such as groceries or suitcases into the car trunk or onto the top shelf of your closet... try using short loop bands around your wrists and elbows when training! Exercising your arms with bands has a series of health benefits which include:

Improved posture: We often think of posture as being something that only affects our appearance but in fact, it affects our physical health too. A poor posture can cause pain in the neck and shoulders, which can lead to headaches and back pain. Exercising your arms will help to build up the muscles in the area so that they are better equipped to support your body weight when you walk upright.

Better balance: The muscles in your arms help maintain balance when standing or walking on uneven surfaces because they provide stability for your body weight. Therefore, exercising these muscles will help improve their strength which will make it easier for you to perform other movements throughout your day. In addition, a stronger upper body means that you will have more control over your movements and be less likely to fall over if you trip or slip. This is especially important as we get older when our balance becomes less stable than it was when we were younger.

Reduced risk of injury: Stronger arm muscles protect us from injury by helping us perform everyday tasks more easily without straining our joints or tendons too much. This allows us to enjoy life without pain or discomfort!

Muscle Tone: Stronger muscles help you maintain a more active lifestyle because they support your body weight better than weak muscles do. When you have strong muscles, they help you to burn calories more quickly throughout the day due to their increased metabolism rate. A combination of strength training arm exercises with aerobic exercises will help you achieve this goal.

Bone Health: As you get older, your bones start to lose their density. This is a natural part of the aging process, but it can be slowed down by strength training. Studies show that those who lift weights tend to lose less bone mass than those who don't. By placing a reasonable amount of stress on your bones, resistance band training can build bone density, which is especially important in later years of life. This in turn can even reduce your risk of developing diseases such as osteoporosis.

Arm strength is a very common term in the world of fitness. It's typically used to refer to how much you can lift or push, but it also refers to how many reps you can do before reaching failure, and how long you can hold something at all. Arm strength is important for almost any activity you can imagine — from driving a car to typing on a computer. The stronger your arms are, the more stable they will be, and the more weight they can hold without fatiguing as quickly.

For your upper arms, there are two primary muscles that you likely know well; the biceps, the triceps and forearms. Biceps consists of two heads: biceps brachii (long head) and biceps brachialis (short head). Both heads work together during elbow flexion and shoulder adduction however the short head is more involved during shoulder extension while both heads are active during pronation/supination (rotating forearm). The biceps brachialis is located on the underside of the upper arm so it's important to train this area.

The triceps make up over two-thirds of the upper arm and are responsible for pushing movements such as bench presses and dips. They are best worked with compound exercises like push-ups but can also be trained by isolation exercises like push-downs.

Forearm muscles. Other than that, there's one often overlooked feature of our arms, even though it makes up for about half of them; our forearms. These are often neglected, but we use them in nearly every functional movement you can name. The forearms are a complex network of muscles, tendons, and ligaments that help us grasp objects and stabilize our wrists for many movements. They're also one of the most neglected areas in the gym, with most people focusing on biceps and triceps instead.

Forearm workouts are a great way to tone your arms. Your forearms are the muscles on the outside of your arm from your elbow to your wrist. They help you pinch, grasp and lift items with more weight than you can manage with just your hands alone. You may want to take a few minutes before exercising to stretch out your wrists, fingers, and forearms so that you do not strain any muscles during exercise.

Forearm workouts are an effective way to build strength and endurance in your hands and arms. They are also a great way to increase hand strength so you can play sports more effectively. Forearm exercises can be done at home with a variety of tools, including hand grippers and wrist weights. You can also do these exercises using your body weight as resistance. There are many ways to strengthen your forearms through exercise, including:

Wrist curls - This is one of the most basic forearm exercises. You simply lift small weights with your wrists, holding the weights close to your body so that only your wrist moves up and down as you curl them up toward your chest then lower them back down again.

Static holds - Static holds work by forcing you to hold on to an object for as long as possible without letting go. For example, try holding onto a barbell or dumbbells with straight arms for 1 minute at a time until you feel like you cannot hold on any longer.

One common way of measuring grip strength is by using a dynamometer (also known as a handgrip dynamometer). You squeeze the handle with all your might until it stops moving; then the device calculates how much force you applied during that period and displays it in pounds or kilograms.

Seniors tend to lose strength in their upper body primarily because they do not strengthen this area as much as other areas, such as the lower body or core area. The loss of muscle mass in your arms can put you at risk for falls because there is less support for your body weight when reaching out. This is why it is important to exercise these areas regularly.

You should exercise your arms at least twice a week. In general, aim for two to three strength-training sessions per week. You could do this by splitting up your workouts into two sessions or by doing one longer session each week. Strength training is important for everyone, but it's especially important for people who want to increase their muscle mass.

If you're new to strength training, start slowly with one or two days per week of exercising your arms. As you get stronger and more comfortable with the exercises, add another day of arm workouts every few weeks until you're up to two or three days per week. Your healthcare provider will be able to design a program for you that meets your needs and goals. Always consult a doctor before starting an exercise program or diet.

When it comes to resistance band exercises for arms, dumbbells are usually the go-to option for most people because they're relatively cheap and easy to store in your home gym closet or under your bed. While dumbbells do have their advantages — namely that they don't roll away when you lay them down — they also have some drawbacks such as being bulky when storing them at home (they take up a lot of space).

Resistance bands on the other hand offer an excellent alternative that is cheaper than traditional dumbbells and takes up less space than free weights. These are 5 great arm exercises you can practice while using resistance bands:

Arm pulls

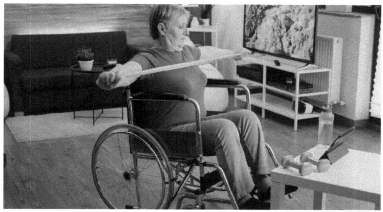

1. Grab your resistance band by both ends and hold it in front of your chest
2. Keep your arms straight with your palms facing down
3. Pull the band sideways
4. During the stretch keep your head and back straight
5. Hold this position for approximately 3 seconds
6. Repeat 5-10 times with 2 sets

Wrist Pulls

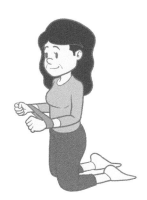

1. Place a short loop band around your wrists
2. Keep your arms in front of you at a 90° angle

3. Keep your back and shoulders straight
4. Pull your arms out
5. Go back to starting position
6. Repeat for 5-8 reps

Y raise

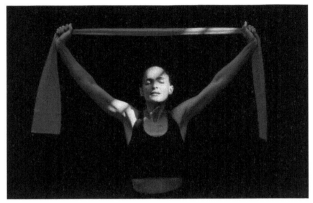

1. Take a long loop or tube band and raise it above your head
2. Keep your back straight and your neck gently tucked
3. Keep your arms straight in a "Y" position
4. Pull the band in both hands until the "Y" is slightly wider
5. Go back to starting position
6. Repeat for 5-8 reps

Side lifts

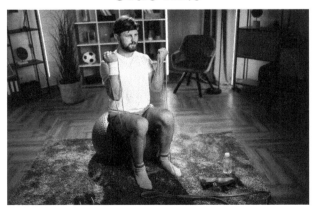

1. Sit down on a chair and place both feet on top of a thera band
2. Grab each side of the band with its corresponding hand
3. Keep arms slightly bent
4. Raise your arms sideways
5. Go back to resting position
6. Repeat for 8-10 reps

Forward pulls

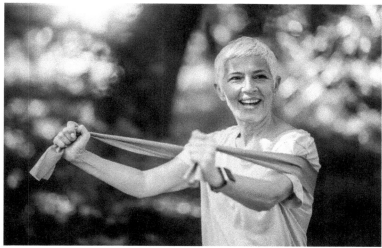

1. Place a thera band around your back
2. Grab each side of the band with its corresponding hand
3. Keep your back straight and your neck gently tucked
4. Keep arms facing up at a 90° angle
5. Pull your hands in front of you until slightly bent
6. Slowly come back to starting position
7. Repeat for 8-10 reps

Arm pullback

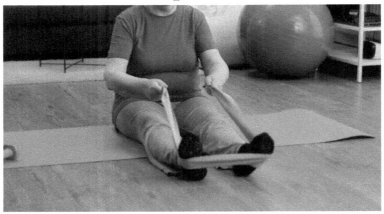

1. Sit on a mat with legs straightened fully
2. Place thera band around your feet and Grab each side of the band with its corresponding hand
3. Keep your legs slightly open and your back straight
4. Keep arms in front of you at a 90° angle
5. Pull band while still keeping your arms at a 90° angle
6. Return to starting position
7. Repeat 8-10 reps

Chapter 8: Leg Exercises

The legs are the largest muscle group in the body, and they're made up of three main muscles — the quadriceps, hamstrings, and glutes. When you work your legs, you are using the largest muscles in your body. This can help you burn a ton of calories and build muscle.

If you want to get fit and stay healthy, it's important to include leg workouts as part of your exercise routine. Leg exercises are an important part of any exercise program, as they help to strengthen your lower body, improve balance and stability, and help to prevent injury.

Leg workouts are often neglected in favor of upper-body workouts, but this is a mistake. Your legs play an important role in helping to support your body weight and reduce the strain on your back and spine.

It's important to maintain strong leg muscles for everyday activities like walking upstairs or getting out of a chair without causing pain or injury. In addition, leg strength helps you perform better in sports that require running or jumping.

The muscles in your lower body are used every time you move your upper body. For example, when you walk or run on the treadmill, you are using all of the muscles in your lower body. When it comes to leg workouts, there are two main types: lower body and upper body. Lower body exercises focus on the muscles surrounding the hip, pelvis, knees, and ankles; these include squats, lunges, and calf raises.

If you have a sedentary lifestyle or suffer from arthritis or other joint pain, leg workouts may be difficult at first. But once you start exercising regularly, your body will adapt and become stronger than it was before.Here are some of the benefits of leg workouts:

Your body needs strong legs if you want to avoid injuries like knee pain or shin splints. Leg workouts can help improve your posture and balance by strengthening your core muscles around your hips and pelvis. These muscles help support the spine so that it doesn't collapse forward under stress (such as when lifting heavy objects). Strengthening them will also improve your overall stability.

Leg workouts are also easier to recover from than upper body workouts because you're using less weight and fewer reps per set. They don't take as much out of your central nervous system as upper body workouts do because you're not pulling the resistance band as much on each set. Here are some reasons why you shouldn't skip leg day:

Improved balance

The legs work together with other muscles in the body to keep us standing up straight and moving forward. This coordination is important for daily activities such as walking or running, but it also helps us perform all types of physical activities like sports or dance. Stronger legs allow us to jump higher and throw farther than people who don't work out their legs regularly!

Build Strength

Leg workouts help build strength in the lower body by working for multiple muscle groups at once in an efficient manner. This includes hamstrings (back of thigh), quadriceps (front of thigh), glutes (buttocks), calves (lower leg), and core muscles like abs and back muscles as stabilizers during exercise movements like squats or lunges for example.

Help prevent osteoporosis

This condition makes it more likely for someone to break a bone. When you work out your legs, this improves the strength of your bones by increasing the amount of density in them. As you age, your body loses more density than it did when you were younger so this is especially important for seniors who are at risk for osteoporosis.

Better Sleep

Leg exercises also help you to sleep better at night because they improve circulation throughout your body. This improves blood flow to your brain so that you can fall asleep faster, stay asleep longer, and wake up feeling more refreshed each morning.

When it comes to exercises, squats are the most rewarding exercises you can do for your lower body — especially if you want strong glutes and thighs! If you've never done squats before but want to start incorporating them into your workout routine, here are a few reasons why they're worth giving a try:

They help build muscle. Squats involve working for multiple large muscle groups at once, which means they're great for building strength and mass. One study found that doing squats for 15 minutes at a fast pace could burn up to 300 calories!

They're easy to incorporate into your routine. You don't have to go to the gym or buy expensive equipment — all you need is an open space and some good music!

If you've never done squats before but want to start incorporating them into your workout routine, here are some of their benefits:

1) Squats help build strong, lean and toned legs.

2) They're a full-body exercise that engages your core, shoulders, and arms along with your lower body.

3) Squats can improve your posture and strengthen your back muscles so you're less likely to develop lower back pain as you age.

4) They improve balance and coordination as well as flexibility in your hips and ankles, which can help prevent injuries while exercising or playing sports.

A few tips to help you improve your leg strength:

Wear compression leggings. Doing so can improve circulation for some people by applying pressure on their legs. This promotes blood flow and supports muscle repair after doing exercises that tone the legs.

Get up from a seated position slowly, especially if you have bad knees or arthritis. If you need help standing up, use a chair or table to assist you with getting up from a seated position. Avoid jumping up to prevent putting too much pressure on your joints. Once you're standing, take at least two steps before sitting back down again — this helps prevent blood pooling in your lower body while sitting down, which can cause clots that lead to deep vein thrombosis (DVT).

Wear shoes that have good arch support and cushioning in the heel. This will help reduce foot pain and fatigue, which can affect your ability to exercise properly.

Start with the lightest bands when doing the exercises as a beginner. Adding too much resistance puts more stress on your muscles and joints than lighter ones do — especially if you haven't used resistance bands before — which can make you feel soreness longer after exercising than if you were using lighter bands.

Rest between sets and workouts so that muscles can recover from being stretched out during exercise sessions. Resting is especially important for people who are new to working out because their bodies need time to strengthen.

When you have a rest day between training sessions, the muscles get stronger as they recover. But if you skip too many workouts in a row, they won't get that chance — and they can start to atrophy instead. It isn't just about losing muscle mass either — if your muscles are too weak when they come back into play again, they could be injured during exercise or in everyday life.

The amount of time between sets is important for building muscle and avoiding injury. When you use resistance bands, your leg fibers tear slightly (this is called microtrauma) and then repair themselves during the rest period between sets. If you don't give yourself enough time for recovery, you risk overtraining and injuring your legs.

Researchers have found that it takes at least 24 hours to 36 hours of rest after working out before your body will respond well to another workout. So if you're strength training two days in a row, there should be at least 48 hours between them. It's also important for beginners to give their bodies an extra day off every week because they recover from exercise more slowly than those who have more experience.

These lower body exercises have been shown to improve balance and stability in seniors who perform them regularly.

Square dance

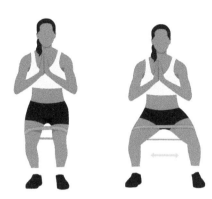

1. Put a short loop band right above the knee
2. Bend knees and open them hip-width while proceeding to stand up straight
3. Place hands on the hips or in front of you
4. Take a step backward with one food and bring the other foot back right after
5. Bring one foot forward and then the other foot forward right after
6. Repeat back and forth several times

For maximum performance try to keep both feet straight and prevent them from turning to the sides too much. It's okay if your feet turn slightly to the side as it is normal for movement. When doing the exercise try to imagine following a square shape when moving your legs back and forth. It is best to do this exercise using two loop bands, one above the knees and one above the ankles. If you do have spare bands lying around then trying this position with two bands will better strengthen your leg area.

Calf pulls

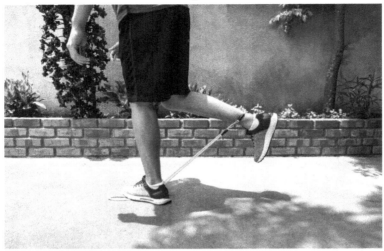

1. Hang on to a chair or a wall for balance
2. Step on one side of a short loop band
3. Place the other leg inside the other end of the loop band
4. Pull the leg upward
5. Slowly go to starting position
6. Repeat for 8-10 reps

Sideway leg raises

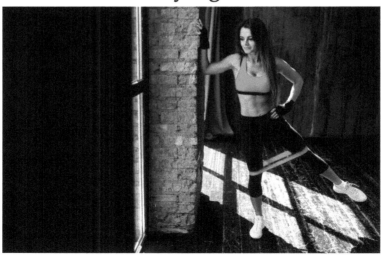

1. Place your arm up against a wall for balance
2. Place a short loop band slightly above ankle level
3. Raise one leg sideways while keeping it straightened out
4. Keep the position for 1 second before returning leg back to the floor
5. Repeat 6-8 times for each leg

Backward leg raises

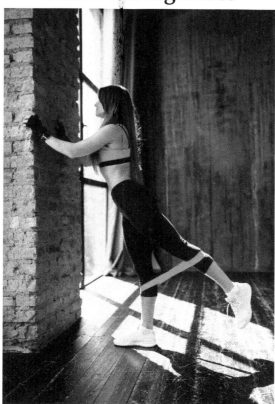

1. Place both arms up against the wall for balance
2. Place a short loop band slightly above ankle level
3. Pull one leg back while keeping it straightened out
4. Keep the position for 1-3 seconds before returning leg on the floor
5. Repeat 6-8 times for each leg

Front crab pulls

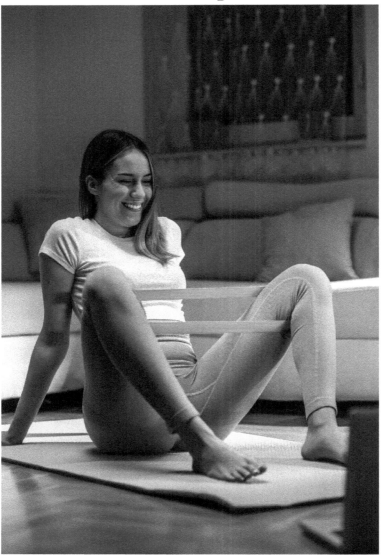

1. Place a short loop band above your knee area
2. Sit down on a yoga mat with legs open at shoulder level
3. Slowly pull sideways with your knees
4. Return to starting position
5. Do 8-10 reps

Side crab pulls

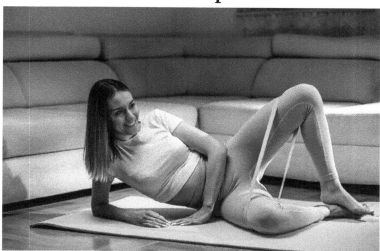

1. Keep the short loop band above your knee area
2. Sit down **SIDEWAYS** on a yoga mat with legs open at shoulder level
3. Slowly raise your leg sideways
4. Return to starting position
5. Do 8-10 reps for each leg

Leg raise

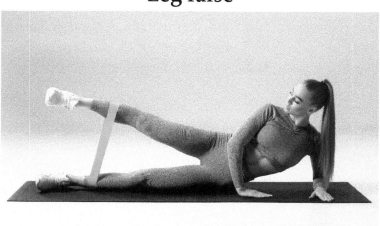

1. Place the short loop band above your ankle area
2. Laydown on a yoga mat with legs fully stretched out
3. Raise leg until you feel resistance (no need to go overboard)
4. Return to starting position
5. Do 8-10 reps for each leg

Chapter 9: Core Work

A strong core is the foundation of a strong body. It's the center of your body, where all movement comes from, and where your power comes from. A strong core helps you maintain good posture while standing or sitting, which leads to better balance. This means less risk of injury during physical activity. It also improves your body mechanics when performing tasks like climbing stairs.

The core includes the lower back, abdomen, and hips (the pelvis). The muscles that make up the core are deep abdominal muscles that stabilize and support the spine, as well as major hip and leg muscles that help with stability and balance.

The core muscles are the main component of a strong core, but other muscles such as the glutes can play a role too. The glutes provide support for your lower back and pelvis, so if those muscles are weak or underdeveloped, it can affect your posture and stability.

Training your core will help improve your overall athleticism and reduce risk factors associated with heart disease, diabetes, and obesity — all of which have been linked to poor muscle tone in this area — according to research published in Medicine & Science in Sports & Exercise in 2010.

In addition to helping improve movement, your core muscles also play an important role in supporting your spine and protecting against back pain. As you age, you may experience some degeneration of these muscles — particularly if you have poor posture or spend long periods sitting at a desk or driving — which can lead to pain and loss of mobility later on.

The core consists of four muscles. These muscles are responsible for trunk stability, spinal mobility, and rotation as well as pelvic stability. They are often referred to as "your belly muscles" because they run around your waistline like a belt that cinches you in tightly from front to back.

These muscles compress the abdomen thus helping to stabilize the lumbar spine during movement by increasing intra-abdominal pressure (pressure inside your abdominal cavity). They also help decrease intra-abdominal pressure during exhalation which allows us to breathe more deeply, promotes proper posture, and supports the proper alignment of our vertebral column during movement.

When these four muscles contract together they allow us to suck in our belly button, lift our rib cage off our pelvis when we inhale, and keep our spine stable while moving our trunk or pelvis in all planes of motion. The deep core muscles have a unique function that is different from other muscles in our body.

They are not meant to move or flex but rather to stabilize the spine and pelvis during the movement of other muscle groups. When we perform exercises such as strengthening exercises, we focus on strengthening these deep core muscles through various movements such as rolls, crunches, side bends, and planks. Strengthening your core has a list of benefits:

Improves flexibility

"The core is the center of stability for our body," says Nicole Albertson, a certified personal trainer and exercise physiologist at the Cleveland Clinic. "If we're not strong in our core, then every time we move, we're going to be relying on our extremities." That means if your core is weak, you'll have to use more energy to move around and pick up objects like groceries and laundry baskets. Plus, you'll have less control over your movements and you will be more likely to injure yourself when lifting weights.

"If you don't engage your core muscles properly while lifting weights or doing resistance exercises (like squats or pushups), then you won't get as much benefit from them," says Albertson. And that means your other muscles won't get as strong either—and neither will the rest of your body!

Increased lifespan

A strong core also helps you live longer. According to the American Council on Exercise (ACE), having a strong core can reduce your risk of chronic diseases such as diabetes, cardiovascular disease, and some cancers. A study published in the Journal of Sports Medicine and Physical Fitness found that core training can reduce your risk of heart disease by lowering blood pressure and improving cholesterol levels. In addition, core training has been shown to improve balance and reduce falls among older adults.

Researchers have also found that a strong core can help prevent osteoporosis by strengthening bones and improving posture. Another study published in the Journal of Strength & Conditioning Research found that women who performed exercises targeting their core had higher bone density than those who didn't.

"We know there's an association between low back pain and decreased physical activity," says Dr. Allison Cieslinski, an orthopedic surgeon at Rush University Medical Center in Chicago. "If you're not moving around enough or doing core exercise, then it's easier for things like arthritis to set in."

Increase stability when participating in sports or other physical activities

A strong core helps you maintain good posture while standing or sitting, which leads to better balance. This means less risk of injury during physical activity such as running. Having a strong core gives you increased functional strength and endurance, which means being able to perform everyday tasks more easily.

Avoid back pain

Core training strengthens the muscles in the abdomen, back, and pelvic floor, which supports the spine and aligns your pelvis in a neutral position so it isn't forced into an anterior tilt (forward tilt). This keeps pressure off the discs between each vertebra, which helps prevent bulging discs from pressing on nerves or causing sciatica pain down your leg.

Ability to breathe easier

The diaphragm is the main muscle for breathing, but if it isn't strong enough to do its job well, you may experience shortness of breath or have trouble sleeping at night because of poor sleep posture (if you're lying on your stomach). Strengthening your core improves diaphragmatic function so you can take deeper breaths without straining yourself.

Have better sexual intercourse

Having a strong core is essential for having good sexual drive! Men who have low testosterone levels may find it difficult to get erections or sustain them during sexual activity if they don't have a strong core. Women may find that they're unable to reach climax unless they have a tight abdominal wall and pelvic floor muscles that contract during these climaxes. A weak core may also cause lower back pain during intercourse due to poor biomechanics or alignment issues such as lordosis (swayback).

But what happens when you have a back injury? Or if you're older and have been living your life sitting down all day long? The answer is that these deep core muscles become inhibited or dysfunctional due to inflammation or poor motor control from years of living an unbalanced lifestyle (i.e., sitting too much). In this case, instead of strengthening these muscles as intended with Pilates or yoga moves, you need to inhibit them further by performing exercises that require too much movement in one direction (i.e., flexion) instead of stabilization.

To understand why these muscles are important for trunk control, we must first review how they work together. When you see a person bend over and touch their toes (without bending at the hips), they will likely have an exaggerated inward curve in their low back (lordosis). This is due to their weak deep core muscles allowing excessive arching of their spine during this movement task.

The deep core muscles also act as a natural shock absorber for your spine. The more toned and strong these muscles are, the better they can support your spine's curvature and keep it upright when you bend over, lift something heavy or jump up on a high step. They also help to prevent back pain by providing support for your back when you stand up straight or bend forward at the waist.

When these muscles become weak or injured they can cause low back pain, SI joint dysfunction (pain), hip issues such as hip bursitis or labral tears, knee pain due to patellar tendonitis (jumper's knee), groin strains/strains/pulls/tears, hamstring strains/strains/pulls/tears and even shoulder impingement syndrome. The best way to keep your body strong and healthy is to perform core exercises at least three times a week. These workouts can be done anytime and anywhere.

Planks are a great way to strengthen your core and improve balance, but they can be challenging. If you're new to planks, start with a knee plank (you'll need a yoga mat or some carpeting) before working up to the full version. "Even if you're in good shape, this exercise can be tough," says Heather Turgeon, an exercise physiologist at the University of New Hampshire. "That's why it's important to build up slowly."

"Planks are one of the best exercises to strengthen your core," says Grant Cohn, owner of Peak Performance Fitness in New York City. "They work on your entire body — all the muscles that stabilize your spine."

The plank is just a static hold in any position that keeps your back straight and your body in a straight line from head to toes. It's a simple exercise, but it requires a lot of focus and concentration. Aside from planks, there are many other core strengthening exercises you can practice while using resistance bands.

Static squat

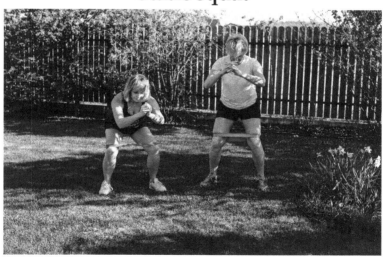

1. Place a short loop band above your knee area
2. Open legs shoulder length
3. Keep back and shoulders straight
4. Take a squat position
5. Make sure your knees don't go in front of your toes
6. Stay in this position for 30 seconds

Russian twists

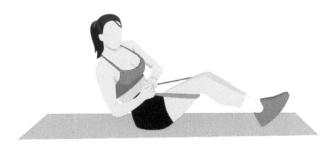

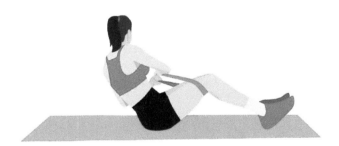

1. Sit on a yoga mat
2. Place a short loop band above your knee area
3. Bend your knees and sit at a 120° angle
4. Keep your feet pointing to the air with your heels touching the ground
5. Grab the band with both hands and twist
6. Twist the body for 15 reps

Core lift

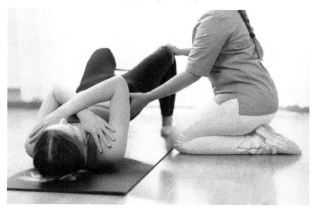

1. Lie down on a yoga mat
2. Place a short loop band above your knee area
3. Keep both arms crossed in front of your chest
4. Move your pelvic area slowly to the top (exhale)
5. Move your pelvic area slowly to the bottom (inhale)
6. Repeat this for 10-15 reps

Side pulls

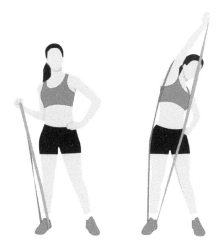

1. Use a long loop band or long thera band
2. Step on one side of the band with one leg and grab the other end with its corresponding hand
3. Keep the same hand with palm facing up and at a 90° angle
4. Raise this hand in a diagonal motion stretching your side core
5. Do this for 8-10 reps for each arm

Abdominal twist

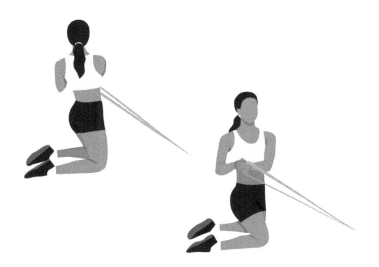

1. Place your resistance band under heavy furniture (table leg)
2. Sit with your knees on the floor and keep the other part of the body straight
3. Grab the other side of the band with both hands
4. Twist your hands along with your core from one side to the other
5. Twist the body for 15 reps

Chapter 10: Moving Forward

There is one crucial element to making a workout effective. This is matching the muscle groups that are being worked. It's not a pretty sight when you're working on your pecs and your shoulders get more of a workout than your chest.

When you're pairing your muscles, you want to make sure that the exercise is taxing them evenly. For example, when pairing your legs with your shoulders, you may wish to do more leg exercises as it's easier for this muscle group to bear more weight than the other. Pairing muscles prevent such a thing from happening.

Pairing muscles is also considered splitting. A split workout is a routine that divides your body into sections, typically upper and lower. Each section of your body is worked on separately, with short rest periods between exercises. Split workouts allow you to focus on one area of the body each day. This can be particularly useful if you want to lose fat while building muscle. There are many ways to structure a split workout, but the most common include:

Full Body Workout - A full body workout trains all of the major muscle groups in a single session. If you are a beginner, then it is recommended only to stick to a full-body workout routine instead of splitting. A splitting workout should be considered only after 6-8 weeks of consistent workout.

A full body workout can be done 2-3 times per week with an emphasis on compound exercises that work multiple muscles at once. Full body workouts are generally performed with lower reps with light to medium resistance and difficulty in order to promote more strength gains than hypertrophy gains.

Upper/Lower Split - An upper/lower split divides your training into two sessions per week where one day focuses primarily on upper body exercises like arms and shoulders, while the other day focuses primarily on lower body exercises such as legs and core. This split allows you to focus more time on each area of your body without fatiguing yourself too much during one session

Push/Pull Split - The push/pull workout splits your body into two parts: pushing muscles and pulling muscles. For example, shoulder day is considered a pushing workout while the core day is considered a pulling workout. This type of split works well because it allows you to work

opposing muscle groups together so you don't get fatigued before your next training session.

Pairing your muscles isn't just about getting more out of your workout; it can also help prevent injury. When you pair large muscle groups together with small ones (for instance, pairing core with arms), you're less likely to over-exert yourself or put too much stress on any one muscle group without giving it enough time to rest between sets. Here is how you can pair muscles during a workout:

Torso (back and chest): These two muscle groups are often paired together because they require similar movement patterns and they both use large amounts of energy during each rep. Some people find it easier to get one workout done in less time by doing these exercises together.

Legs and Arms: The quadriceps (front of the thigh) and hamstrings (back of the thigh) are also best paired together. This is because both are used to produce force during exercise, although they have different functions. For example, the quadriceps work with your glutes to extend your leg forward from a bent position (i.e., knee extension), while the hamstrings pull your leg backward from a straightened position (i.e., knee flexion). Since these movements involve opposing muscle groups working together, you can think of them as a pair that should be worked out at the same time or close together to avoid overtraining or possible injury.

Shoulders and upper torso (chest): Shoulders and upper torso exercises have a lot in common — many of them require you to raise your arms above your head or forward from your body. The front side of your body is generally worked more during chest exercises, while the back side is worked more during shoulder exercises. However, many chest exercises will involve some sort of pushing motion for the shoulders and vice versa.

Back/Biceps: This pairing is a classic weight training combination because these two muscle groups work together during many different exercises such as pull-ups or chin-ups and bicep curls. It's not only possible but also recommended that you pair back exercises with biceps exercises when building muscle mass in this area. This is because when you do a biceps curl or row, you'll be using some of the muscles in your back as well.

Resting

When you work out, your muscle fibers become damaged and sore. Your body needs time to repair this damage, so it can strengthen the muscles and prevent future injuries. If you don't give your body this time to recover, you could end up overtraining and injuring yourself or even wearing down your muscles so much that they stop functioning properly.

Rest days are important for mental health as well. Exercise helps relieve stress by releasing endorphins into the bloodstream, but if you never take time off, this can lead to burnout and even depression. Rest days also give your mind a chance to relax and recharge so that it's ready for another workout session later on.

On rest days, you should still get some physical activity — such as walking or stretching — but avoid strenuous exercise or other activities that would be stressful on your body. You should also take care not to overexert yourself on your rest days; otherwise, you risk getting injured or overtrained.

The purpose of resting is to give your body time to repair itself after workouts. The more intense the workout, the longer it will take your body to recover. For example, if you're running several miles every other day, then you'll probably need at least two full days off each week to allow your muscles time to rebuild themselves before they can handle another challenging run session. A rest day is a perfect way to recharge your batteries, but it can be hard to tell if a person needs one. Here are some signs to look out for:

You're getting sick. Tiredness is often the first sign of illness. If you're feeling run down, it's probably best to take a break and let your body recover.

You can't remember what it feels like to be pain-free. If you're always in pain, this may mean that your body needs a break from whatever activity you're doing. This could mean taking more frequent breaks and stretching during long periods of sitting.

Struggling with concentration or memory problems. Focus and memory are linked with sleep quality; if someone is struggling with either of these things, they may need more sleep than usual or they may need a rest day so they can get better quality sleep at night (if they're getting enough sleep).

You wake up feeling sore every morning. If waking up with sore muscles is common for you, then this may be an indication that you need to take more rest days or reduce your physical activity levels. Soreness can also be caused by muscle imbalances — when one muscle group is stronger than another — if this might be an issue for you, get it corrected by working with a physical therapist who can prescribe exercises to help correct imbalances in muscle groups and improve joint mobility for greater comfort during movement.

You are constantly hungry (or thirsty). Hunger and thirst are both signs that your body needs food and water to function properly. If you find yourself constantly hungry, it could mean that you are over exercising and need to rest for your body to regain back energy.

Diet

Seniors can have trouble absorbing nutrients because their bodies are less able to use them. They are more prone to have medical conditions that affect their nutrition in comparison with the general population. Some reasons seniors have trouble maintaining a proper diet are:

Changes in taste and smell. Your sense of taste and smell may decline with age, which can reduce your enjoyment of foods. This can make it harder for you to notice when food is past its prime or spoiled.

Changes in digestion. As we get older, our bodies don't work as well at digesting certain nutrients and vitamins from food. This means that older adults need fewer calories than younger adults do in order to maintain their weight and avoid gaining weight as they age.

Changes in appetite. Older people often have smaller appetites than younger people do, even if they're not sick or frail. They also tend to eat less at meals than younger people do because they're less likely to be hungry between meals or late at night when they sleep.

Changes in the body's ability to absorb nutrients from food. The body's ability to absorb nutrients from food depends on several factors, such as how much vitamin B12 is stored in the liver and how much iron is stored in the blood.

Getting the right amount of nutrients is crucial for good health. But it can be difficult to get all the nutrients you need from food alone. If you're older or have certain health conditions, it's even more important to make sure you're getting enough vitamins and minerals each day.

The best way to make sure you're getting enough vitamins and minerals is by eating a variety of foods so that you get all the nutrients you need. A healthy diet includes plenty of fruits and vegetables, whole grains (such as brown rice), and legumes (such as beans). It also includes lean meats like fish or poultry; low-fat dairy products such as cheese or yogurt; and nuts and seeds in moderation because they are high in fat.

Older adults should also limit their intake of saturated fats (found mostly in animal products such as red meats) because these fats tend to increase blood cholesterol levels over time. In fact, a healthy diet is one of the best things you can do to maintain your health as you get older. The following sections discuss some key nutrients that are especially important for seniors and how to get enough of them in your diet. If you follow these steps, you can help keep yourself healthy:

Don't eat empty calories. Foods with empty calories are low in nutrients— such as chips, candy, and baked goods. They don't provide much nutrition for their calories so they're often called "junk food." If you do eat junk food occasionally, make sure it's not the main part of your meal or snack.

Take calcium and Vitamin D. Calcium is necessary for strong bones and teeth. It helps keep your bones strong so they don't break easily. It also helps prevent tooth decay by promoting remineralization (the process of rebuilding minerals on the surface of teeth).

Vitamin D helps with calcium absorption and bone health by increasing calcium stores in the body's soft tissues (including muscle) rather than just in the bones themselves. Vitamin D deficiency has been linked to osteoporosis and other bone diseases such as osteomalacia in older adults. The best way to get enough calcium is through food — not supplements — because foods provide other nutrients that work together with calcium.

Choose lean proteins, such as skinless chicken breast, or fish such as salmon or tuna, instead of red meat. Lean proteins provide many vitamins and minerals that contribute to good health in older adults. If you have trouble getting enough protein, you can use protein supplements such as powder shakes made with soy milk or other non-dairy milk. Or try adding a few nuts or seeds to your diet.

Choose whole grains over refined grains. Whole grains are high in fiber, which helps keep you full throughout the day, and they can help lower cholesterol levels and blood sugar levels—both risk factors for heart disease. They also have more vitamins and minerals than refined grains do, such as iron and magnesium (which helps control blood pressure). The best sources of whole grains include: 100 percent whole wheat bread or pasta; brown rice; quinoa; oatmeal; popcorn; and whole grain cereal (check nutrition labels to be sure it's 100 percent whole grain).

Eat plenty of fruits and vegetables. They're rich in vitamins A, C, and E; folate; potassium; iron; calcium; magnesium; carotenoids (plant pigments); flavonoids (antioxidants); lutein/zeaxanthin (which protect against eye diseases); lycopene (which protects against prostate cancer); selenium; omega-3 fatty acids (which protect brain function); zinc; chromium (which helps regulate blood sugar); copper; manganese and molybdenum (which help synthesize amino acids).

Drink plenty of water daily. About eight glasses for women and 10 for men — to keep your body hydrated throughout the day. Water is important because it carries nutrients to your cells and gets rid of waste products from your body. It also helps control blood pressure and body temperature.

Cut back on saturated fats (such as butter) by using olive oil instead on salads or in cooking when possible. Saturated fats raise cholesterol levels in your blood which increases your risk of heart disease.

Reduce sodium intake. Sodium is linked to high blood pressure, which increases your risk of heart disease, stroke, and kidney disease. To lower your sodium intake at home, look for low-sodium varieties of canned soups, low-sodium broths,and low-sugar ketchup at the grocery store or supermarket.

Choose low-fat or nonfat dairy products. Low-fat or nonfat dairy products are good sources of calcium and vitamin D, which are important for keeping bones strong as you age. Choose skim milk rather than 2% or whole milk when possible; it contains slightly less fat but still provides most of the nutrients found in whole milk — including calcium. You can also try soy milk or almond milk as an alternative to regular milk if you're trying to limit your intake of animal proteins like meat or eggs (which can be high in saturated fats).

Eat smaller portions. One of the biggest challenges for older adults is eating too much food at once. It's important to slow down and take time to chew your food well. This helps prevent choking and allows your body time to digest it properly. It's also a good idea to avoid eating right before bed because this can cause heartburn or indigestion if you sleep with a full stomach. Your body needs at least three hours after eating before bedtime so it has time to process all the food before sleep.

Keep a food diary to help you identify foods that trigger cravings. You might find that certain foods make you feel sick after eating them, or that they don't fill you up as much as others. If so, try to avoid those foods in your diet.

If necessary, ask your doctor about medication that may help calm or increase your appetite by boosting serotonin levels in the brain. Other medications can also be helpful for some people, such as those with diabetes or high blood pressure.

Training experience is always a debate surrounding exercise. The more you do it the better you get at it and make it look easy to an untrained eye. So more advanced movements should be easier than what we first attempt, right? That's true in some situations. But how much easier do we really want our exercises to be?

1. When Should You Modify Exercises?

If you have any pain or injuries in your joints or muscles, it's best to modify exercises that put pressure on these areas. For example, if you have knee pain, avoid lunges and squatting movements; if you have shoulder pain, avoid pushing movements; if you have wrist pain, avoid bicep curls and push-ups; etc.

2. What Should You Modify?

If there are certain parts of an exercise that are uncomfortable for you to perform — especially when compared to other people you are working out with— then it's time to modify it! For example: If you can only do 10 second planks but everyone else is doing 30 (or more!), then it might be time to modify it by putting your knees down.

3. Is the Exercise Safe?

Some exercises may be unsafe for certain people. For example, if you have knee pain, then you shouldn't perform squats because they put a lot of stress on your knees. To start slow and grow with time, you are free to follow this 12-week workout routine (note that the instructions for how to perform the exercises and the number of reps were covered earlier in the book).

Stretching

Stretching is often used as a warm-up for physical activities, such as running and resistance training, or as an injury prevention measure.

It can also be used to improve the flexibility of muscles, tendons, and joints in order to reduce the potential damage that may be caused by the shortening of these tissues during a workout. Stretches are performed before or after exercise, or at any other time when muscles are cold and tight.

And it is not just for people who want flexible joints; it can help with overall health. Many people who suffer from stiff muscles and joints are able to enjoy pain relief through regular stretching exercises.

A recent study found that stretching before exercise can decrease the risk of injuries among runners by up to 50 percent. Many people think that stretching is simply yoga. But there's a lot more to it than that.

Yoga and stretching are related, but they're not the same thing. Yoga is a system of exercise and meditation. It has its roots in religion, but people don't need to be religious to do it.

Stretching on the other hand, is a way of improving flexibility by holding poses for longer periods of time or by adding resistance (such as weights or bands) to your body parts.

Yoga focuses on developing strength and flexibility through postures (called asanas) and breathing techniques (called pranayama). The goal of yoga isn't just to improve flexibility; it's also about calming your mind and improving balance, endurance, and mental focus — all things that will help you perform better in sports and other activities where you need strong muscles along with good coordination and mental focus.

Unlike yoga, stretching is a crucial part of any workout routine. It not only helps you to avoid injury and improves your range of motion, but it also helps the body warm up for exercise. Warming up increases blood flow to the muscles, which means that there's more oxygen and nutrients available for your muscles to use during exercise.

It also helps to loosen the muscles, which improves their elasticity and reduces the risk of injury. The best way to stretch is to hold each position for 10 to 15 seconds before repeating on the other side. You should feel a slight pull in your muscles without experiencing pain. Don't bounce or strain against the stretch — just allow gravity to do its job! Here are some of the most common stretches you can do before a workout:

Quadriceps stretch

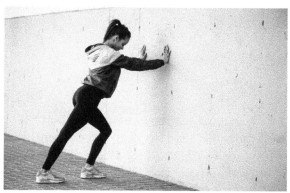

Stand facing a wall with both feet flat on the floor and about an inch away from it. Lower your upper body toward the wall until you feel a stretch in your front thigh muscle (the quadriceps). Hold for 20 seconds, then relax. Repeat three times on each leg.

Hamstring stretch

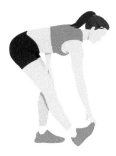

Stand with one foot forward and one foot back (or sit on a chair), keeping both knees slightly bent so that your lower back doesn't arch too much in either direction (a sign of poor form). Slowly bend from your hips toward the floor until you feel the tension in your hamstrings. Hold for 20 seconds, then relax.

Sitting extension stretch

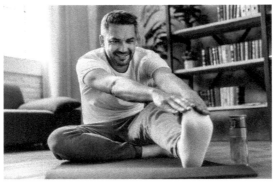

Sit on the floor with one leg extended straight out in front of you and the other bent with your foot flat on the floor. Pull your toes toward you, then push them away from you until you feel a stretch in the front of your thigh. Hold for 30 seconds, then switch legs and repeat.

Calf stretch

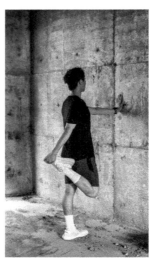

Stand facing a wall with both feet approximately 12 inches away from it and parallel to each other. Rest one hand on the wall while bending one leg behind you so that your heel is touching the wall. Lean forward until you feel a gentle stretch in your calves. Hold for 10 seconds, then switch legs and repeat 3 times per leg.

Stretching after a workout is especially important because it helps to relax the body and muscles. After exercise, your body releases endorphins, which are natural painkillers that make you feel good. When you stretch after a workout, these endorphins remain in the bloodstream longer than if you had not stretched at all.

Stretching helps to increase blood flow to all parts of the body. This improves circulation and helps remove lactic acid from your muscles, which reduces soreness after exercise. A warm muscle has more blood vessels open, allowing more blood to flow through it. This means that more oxygen is delivered to working muscles and nutrients are delivered to damaged muscle fibers.

As you stretch, your body releases chemicals called endorphins — also known as painkillers — and other hormones that relieve stress and reduce anxiety. Stretching can also help you relax after a stressful day or bring about sleepiness if done before bedtime.

But be aware that it can cause injury if you do too much too quickly or if you have an underlying medical condition such as arthritis or fibromyalgia (a disorder characterized by widespread musculoskeletal pain and tenderness). If you're not sure how much stretching is right for you, talk with your doctor first. The most common post workout stretching positions are the cobra stretch and the child pose as they prove to be more effective on your upper body. You can also, however, practice these three other stretches for the lower body after your workout:

Butterfly

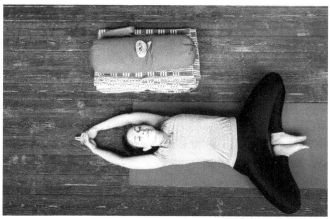

To perform the butterfly, lie on your back with your knees bent and feet flat on the floor. Bring your hands over your head. Bend both feet and move them as close as possible to your groin area until you feel a stretch in your inner thighs; hold for 30 seconds then let go.

Standing Quadricep Stretch

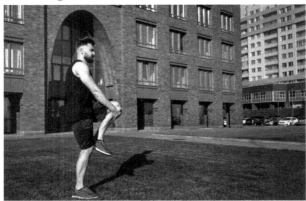

Begin this quadriceps (in the front of the thigh) by standing with legs slightly open. Bend your right leg and hold on to the foot in front of your chest, keeping weight on the heel. Straighten the leg in front of you and keep the back straight. Hold for 20 to 30 seconds, then repeat on the other side.

Seated Spinal Twist

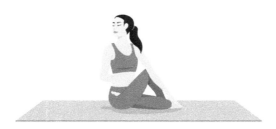

This is another great pose for beginners. You can do this pose seated on the floor or in a chair if you're more comfortable with your back supported. Sit up tall with your legs crossed in front of you and your feet about hip-width apart. Place your right hand behind your right leg and turn towards it until you feel a stretch through your left side. Take this time to breathe deeply into the stretch. Repeat on the other side.

12-week beginners resistance band workout

NOTE: For the best results always exhale while doing the workout and inhale when going back to the starting position.

Exercise Time: 15 - 20 minutes per session

Exercise volume: 4 days a week

Woodchopper

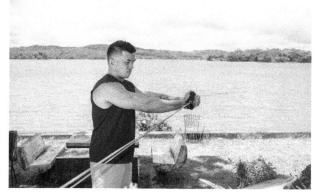

To do this exercise, hold both ends of the resistance band with the corresponding hand and stand with feet shoulder-width apart and knees slightly bent. Bring one end of the band up to chest level while twisting at the hips to bring in the opposite side (the other end) behind you. You should feel tension on your obliques as you twist. Then bring it back down to chest level and repeat for 2 reps before switching sides.

Triceps kickbacks

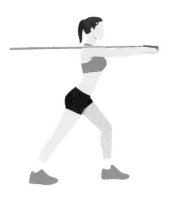

Stand facing away from the anchor point of the resistance band, holding it with both hands in front of your body at chest level. Your palms should be facing inward towards each other. Bend both elbows 90 degrees so that they are at right angles with your upper arms, then slowly straighten them back out again until they're fully extended but not locked out (this will be about 45 degrees). When performing this exercise, make sure that you don't allow your elbows to come together behind your body as this will cause unnecessary stress on them and could lead to injury.

Pull-apart exercise

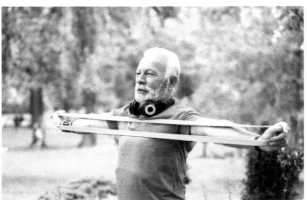

This is a great exercise for developing shoulders and arms. To do it, stand up and keep your legs slightly apart and knees slightly bent. Hold one end of the band in the corresponding hand so that it's taut and there's no slack in the middle. Bring your hands together so that they're touching at chest level with palms facing each other. Then slowly pull them apart until they are at ear level with palms facing away from you at all times.

Overhead pull-apart

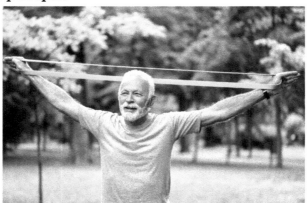

Stand facing with your feet together and knees slightly bent. Grab both ends of the band with one hand on each handle and raise them up overhead until both arms are extended straight above you. Slowly pull the handles apart while keeping your arms straight overhead. Once they're fully stretched out overhead, slowly return them to their original position above your head. Repeat this 8-10 times for one set and perform 3-4 sets total.

Bicep curl

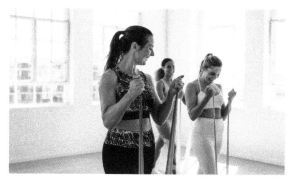

Stand with feet hip-width apart, knees slightly bent, and back straight. Hold the center of a resistance band in each hand, palms facing down with wrists bent back and elbows slightly bent. Arms should be extended out in front of you (you may have to adjust your grip on the band as you progress). Squeeze your shoulder blades together as you bring your hands toward your shoulders until they almost touch behind you. Slowly return to the starting position.

Bent-over row

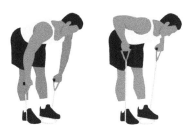

To perform this exercise, stand straight with your legs slightly open and hold the band in both hands with your arms extended at chest height. Your palms should be facing down and your elbows should be bent at 90 degrees. Slowly pull the band towards your chest by bending at the waist until you feel a stretch in your shoulders, then slowly return to starting position. Repeat for eight to 12 repetitions.

Standing side taps

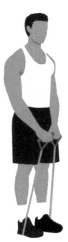
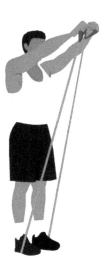

Start by standing with your feet together, holding the band in both hands. Squeeze your shoulder blades together and hold the band with your arms straight out in front of you at chest level. Pull the band over your head, keeping your legs straight and knees locked. Return to the starting position and repeat 10 times.

Overhead press

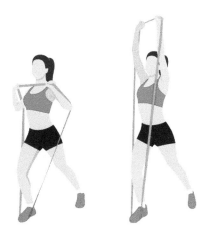

Start with one foot forward, standing on top of the band, and the other foot back behind you. Switch your grip, grabbing the handles from underneath so that your palms are facing forward and away from you. Start by holding the handles at shoulder height. Then add pressure over your head, extending both arms straight above you. Repeat 8-10 times.

Standing lateral band walk

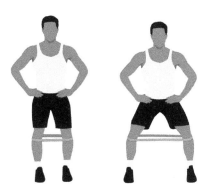

Place feet in a resistance band with both feet slightly open. Grab the hips and slightly bend your body so that you feel the tension in the band. Keep your back straight and shoulders down as you rotate your hips outward. Now open one leg outward and then step inward with that same leg until both feet are together again. That's one rep! Repeat for 8 reps per side before switching legs and repeating again for an additional 8 reps per side.

Standing banded squat

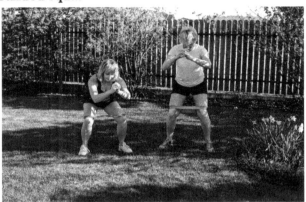

This is a great exercise to start with, as it's simple and easy to do. Simply wrap the band around your knees You can then squat down and stand up again while keeping the tension in the band. You can also do this exercise while holding on to a chair if you have balance issues, just make sure to keep your knee soft! This exercise will help improve your core stability, which makes it a great addition to any workout routine.

Banded bridge

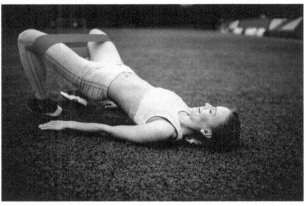

To do this exercise, place a resistance band around your hips and lie on your back with your knees bent and feet flat on the floor. Then squeeze your glutes and drive through your heels as you press up into a bridge position. Hold for one count at the top of the movement before lowering back down to starting position. If you're using an extra-thick band, you'll need to make sure it's anchored securely so it doesn't slip or slide off during your set. If you're using a lighter band, try using two hands to anchor the band so it doesn't slip or slide off during your set.

Intermediate: Week 4 - 12+

In weeks 9 -12+, you will do a split workout.

NOTE: For the best results always exhale while doing the workout and inhale when going back to the starting position.

Exercise Time: 15 - 20 minutes per session

Exercise volume: 5 days a week

NOTE: Do 3 full body workouts and 2 split workout sessions a week.

Arm & Leg Day
Overhead Pull-Apart

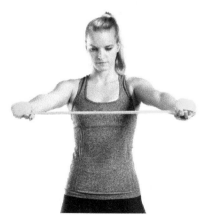

The overhead pull-apart is similar to the push-up, but you're using resistance bands instead of body weight to challenge your body even further. To perform this exercise, hold the band with both hands above your head and pull.

Front Raise

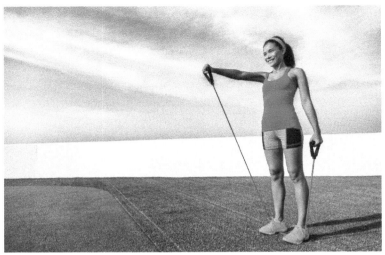

Stand with your feet shoulder-width apart and hold the ends of the resistance band. With your arms bent at 90 degrees and palms facing forward, raise your one arm out in front of you until it is parallel to the floor. Your elbows should be flexed at 90° and your forearms should be vertical throughout the exercise. Slowly return to the starting position and repeat for desired reps on both arms.

Pull-Apart

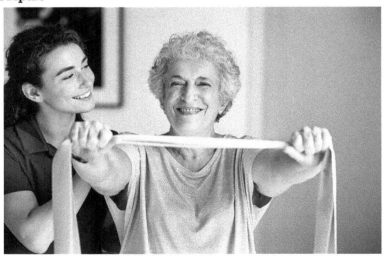

This is a great exercise to work your back and shoulders. The key to this exercise is to not just go through the motions but really focus on squeezing those muscles. It's also important to keep your back straight and your shoulders down and away from your ears.

Bent-Over T Flies

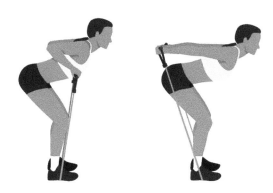

To perform this exercise, start by holding the handles of the resistance band. Bend over at the hips and keep your back straight. Your arms should be bent down from your shoulders with palms facing forward. Now raise your arms back until they are almost parallel to the floor. You should feel this in your chest and upper back. Lower your arms back down to starting position and repeat for reps or time.

Leg Lifts

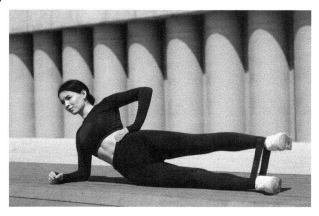

Put a resistance band around both ankles while lying sideways on the floor. Lift your right leg up as high as possible without straining. Hold for two seconds then slowly lower your leg down to the starting position. Repeat this movement with your other leg. Perform three sets of 15 reps on each side.

Squats

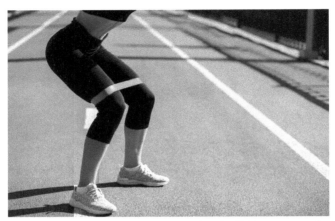

The squat is one of the best exercises for building strength and muscle mass. It works your entire lower body, and it's particularly effective for targeting your glutes, quads, and hamstrings. By adding a resistance band to this exercise, you can increase the intensity of the movement while also improving your balance and stability. Do 8-10 reps for 2 sets.

Lateral Band Walk

LATERAL STEPS & SQUATS
WITH RESISTANCE BAND

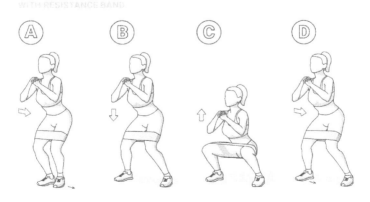

This is an effective way to work on lateral stability, which is important for good posture and preventing injury. Stand with your feet together and the band wrapped around your thighs. Step out to the right with your other leg,and follow with the other. Slowly move sideways while slightly squatting until you feel a moderate stretch on the outside of your right thigh. Hold for two seconds for each full step you take, then step back to the center with both feet. Repeat this movement 10 times.

Glute Kickbacks

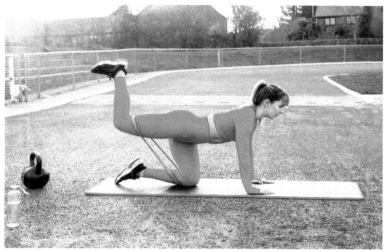

The gluteus maximus is a large muscle that makes up the buttocks. This exercise targets the glutes while building strength in the hamstrings and lower back.

With all fours on a mat, place a resistance band placed at knee level. Keep your arms straight and one leg on the floor while raising the other leg. The resistance band should be pulled tight, so you feel the tension in your glutes when you kick back.

Keeping your chest lifted and core engaged, kick back one leg at a time as far as you can, then return to starting position by extending your leg behind you without locking out your knee. Focus on keeping your hips square and not arching or leaning forward. Perform 10 reps on each side before moving on to the next exercise.

Shoulders & Back Day

Side raises

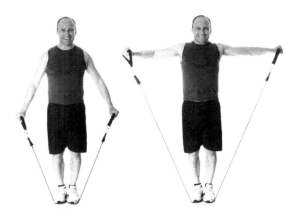

Hold resistance bands with both hands, palms facing your body. Raise your arms outwards until they are parallel to the floor, keeping them at shoulder height. Slowly lower your arms back down to starting position. Repeat 15 times on both sides.

Upright row

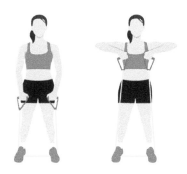

Grasp the handles of the band, holding them with both hands at waist level and slightly wider than shoulder-width apart. Position your arms straight out with elbows bent 90 degrees. Your palms should be facing each other. Now raise both arms up towards the ceiling until they are almost pointing to the ground while keeping your elbows slightly bent. Return to starting position and repeat for 10 to 12 repetitions with both arms.

Bent-over rows

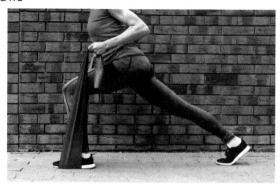

To perform bent-over rows with a resistance band, stand with your feet apart and hold one end of the band with the corresponding hand at arm's length in front of your body. Keep your elbows close to your sides as you bend forward at the waist until it feels like you're about to lose balance. Place one foot forward and the other foot behind you.

Step on the band with the foot that you placed forward, then pull the band up toward your chest while keeping elbows close to the sides (you should feel this in your back muscles). Reverse movement back down until arms are straight out again.

Straight-arm pulldown

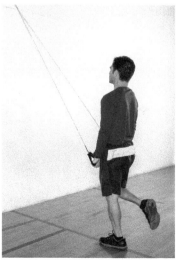

Attach the long tube band to a door or anchor on the wall, making sure it is secure. While standing up, maintain the same distance between your arms and torso throughout the movement. Slowly pull the handles of the band down toward your side until it touches your hip before returning to the start position. Repeat with the opposite arm to complete one rep.

Full Body 2x

One-arm biceps curl

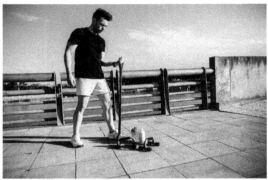

Stand with your legs slightly apart, knees slightly bent, hold the resistance band with your right hand and step on the other side of the band with your right leg. This is your starting position. Then raise your right arm up in front of you until it's parallel to the floor. Slowly return to the starting position and repeat on the other side.

Side-lying hip abduction

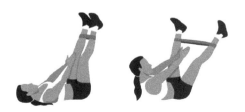

Lie on your side with your legs in the air out in front of you, knees slightly bent, and feet together. Wrap the band around both legs just above your ankles, then pull your legs apart as much as your body allows you to. Keep your core engaged, and abs are drawn in as you keep your legs lifted. You should feel this in your outer thighs. Repeat on both sides until you've completed 5-8 reps per side.

Wall squat

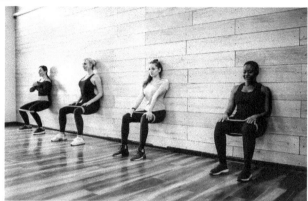

Attach the resistance band around your ankles, knees, or thighs. The higher up you attach it, the more difficult the exercise will be. Rest your back against a wall and take a squat position. Keep your core tight and chest up as you hinge at the hips and bend forward at the waist until your buttocks are parallel to the floor. Hold this position for 5 counts before returning to standing. Repeat 2 times.

Splitter

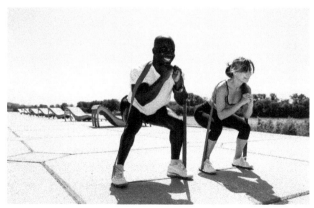

To do this exercise, you will need a long band. The wider the band, the easier it is to do this exercise. Set up in a split stance with your feet apart at least as wide as your shoulders. Step on the band and secure the other end above your shoulders. Your elbows should be bent slightly and pointing out to the side with palms facing forward or up toward the ceiling at about shoulder height.

Step forward into a squat position, keeping knees bent 90 degrees or less with both feet on the floor. Return to starting position by straightening the elbows back out in front of the body while stepping back into starting position. Repeat this motion until you have completed 5 reps per side.

Glute bridge

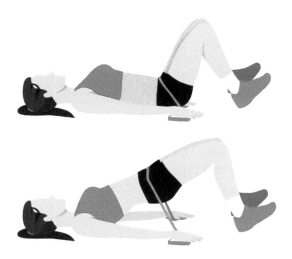

Start lying on your back with your feet flat on the floor and your knees bent at 90 degrees, holding onto each end of the resistance band with both hands. Your arms should be extended while holding the band across your pelvic area (depending on how much weight you want to use). Press through your heels into the floor as you squeeze your glutes together to lift your hips off the ground until they form a straight line from knees to shoulders. Pause for 2 seconds at the top of the movement before lowering back down slowly until your butt touches the ground again.

Squat to overhead press

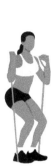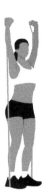

Go down into a squat, keeping our head up. And then come back up and press over your head with the band. As you come back down, push out at the bottom of the squat so that you get some good extension at the top of your range of motion. Make sure to keep your hips straight down and not moving side-to-side as well. So keep your heels flat on the ground and push out at the bottom of the squat for a great posterior chain exercise using resistance bands!

Lateral walk/steps

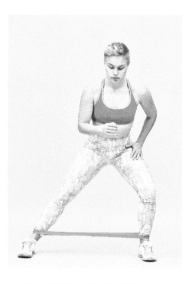

This exercise helps strengthen the muscles on both sides of your body. It also helps in improving balance while walking, running, or jogging. To do this exercise, stand straight with feet hip-width apart, and bend one knee while keeping the other foot flat on the ground. Walk sideways with one foot at a time while keeping the knee raised up all throughout the motion. Do 10-12 repetitions with each leg before switching sides.

Strive for success

The more you live your life, the more you realize that there are so many opportunities to do something different and make a change. The first thing you need to do is develop a positive attitude.

This is the foundation of all confidence-building activities. Being aware of your emotions and thoughts is important because they can affect your actions. For example, if you are feeling sad or depressed, it will be hard for you to get up and start doing your daily workout session.

So, to build self-confidence, you need to start by changing your thoughts and feelings about yourself. When you think positively about yourself and your abilities, you will find it easier to take action towards achieving your goals.

Another thing that helps with gaining self-confidence is having a strong sense of fulfillment in life. Seniors who have this kind of fulfillment tend to be happier and more resilient when faced with challenges or setbacks because they are driven by something greater than themselves, such as family, religion, or community service work. There are many ways to gain the right confidence and accomplish your exercise goals. Here are a few suggestions:

1. Set goals for yourself that you want to achieve by keeping a daily journal. For example, if you want to gain muscle, list the steps that need to be taken to reach your goal, and then check them off as they are completed. This will help keep you focused on your goal and also give you a sense of accomplishment when each step is completed. Write how you felt for the day and whether you exercised or not. Journaling

significantly increases your chances of success.

2. If you have ever done something difficult or challenging but ultimately rewarding (e.g., finally completing 30-second plank), think back on that experience and remember how proud you felt once you had accomplished it. Try to recapture those feelings by thinking about what it was like when you first started learning to do something new and difficult. However, you knew deep down inside that you would eventually succeed because you always do what's best for yourself!

3. Start doing things on your own without relying on others so much for help, advice, or reassurance (e.g., asking a friend what they think before starting your exercise journey). Once we practice doing this enough, we'll become more confident in our abilities without the need for constant validation. This tip doesn't count for your doctor or healthcare provider, as you should always ask them for help or advice when needed.

The first step to succeeding in this new journey is overcoming mental barriers. The key is to focus on the end result. Do your best to ignore what other people think about seniors gaining muscle by pulling some bands around. Instead, focus on becoming the best and healthiest version of yourself.

The benefits of exercising with resistance bands are numerous, but most importantly, it can help you live a longer and healthier life. Working out improves cardiovascular health, reduces stress, and promotes better sleep habits. When it comes to exercise, age is just a number.

"The biggest challenge is mental," says Dr. Andrew Hunt, a sports medicine physician who coaches cross-country runners (Brigham and Women's Hospital in Boston). "You have to overcome everything telling you not to do it."

Hunt says he sees this every year with his runners – many of whom are beginners when they start training for cross-country in September. They go through several phases before learning how to run properly – starting with walking and then building up their endurance over weeks or months until they can run for longer periods without stopping for rest breaks or pain relief medication like ibuprofen or acetaminophen.

Eating healthy and exercising more often is often much easier said than done. Many people have had bad experiences with diets and workouts because it all starts with the mind. Getting up from the couch and going for a workout can feel more daunting than it should. It takes more than just motivation to get yourself in good shape; it also requires mental strength and discipline.

The best way to overcome these mental barriers is to start by focusing on what you need to do daily. Take it one day at a time. *Don't get discouraged.*

Here's another book by Scott Hamrick that you might like

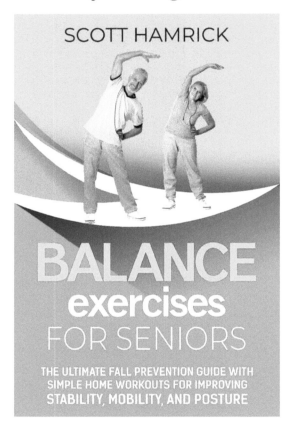

Free Bonuses from Scott Hamrick

Hi seniors!

My name is Scott Hamrick, and first off, I want to THANK YOU for reading my book.

Now you have a chance to join my exclusive "workout for seniors" email list so you can get the ebook below for free as well as the potential to get more ebooks for seniors for free! Simply click the link below to join.

P.S. Remember that it's 100% free to join the list.

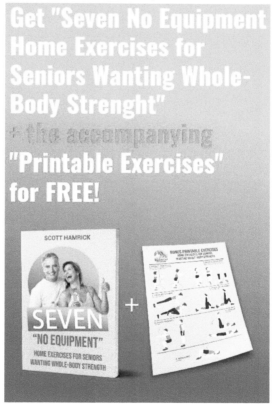

Access your free bonuses here
https://livetolearn.lpages.co/strength-training-for-seniors-paperback1/

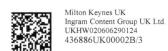

Milton Keynes UK
Ingram Content Group UK Ltd.
UKHW020606290124
436886UK00002B/3